Coconut Oil for Health

100 Amazing and Unexpected Uses for Coconut Oil

Britt Brandon, CFNS, CPT

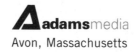
Aadamsmedia
Avon, Massachusetts

Published by
Adams Media, a division of F+W Media, Inc.
57 Littlefield Street, Avon, MA 02322. U.S.A.
www.adamsmedia.com

Contains material adapted and abridged from *The Everything® Coconut Diet Cookbook* by Anji Sandage,
copyright © 2012 by F+W Media, Inc, ISBN 10: 1-4405-2902-7, ISBN 13: 978-1-4405-2902-3.

ISBN 10: 1-4405-8591-1
ISBN 13: 978-1-4405-8591-3
eISBN 10: 1-4405-8592-X
eISBN 13: 978-1-4405-8592-0

Printed in the United States of America.

10   9   8   7   6   5   4   3   2   1

Library of Congress Cataloging-in-Publication Data

Brandon, Britt.
  Coconut oil for health / Britt Brandon, CFNS, CPT.
     pages cm
  Includes index.
  ISBN 978-1-4405-8591-3 (pb) -- ISBN 1-4405-8591-1 (pb) -- ISBN 978-1-4405-8592-0 (ebook) -- ISBN 1-4405-8592-X
(ebook)
  1. Coconut oil--Health aspects. 2. Coconut oil--Therapeutic use. 3. Fatty acids in human nutrition. 4. Beauty, Personal. I.
Title.
  QP144.O44B73 2015
  664'.36--dc23
                                    2014038757

Many of the designations used by manufacturers and sellers to distinguish their products are claimed as trademarks. Where those designations appear in this book and F+W Media, Inc. was aware of a trademark claim, the designations have been printed with initial capital letters

The various uses of coconut oil as a health aid are based on tradition, scientific theories, or limited research. They often have not been thoroughly tested on humans, and safety and effectiveness have not yet been proven in clinical trials. Some of the conditions for which coconut oil can be used as a treatment or remedy are potentially serious, and should be evaluated by a qualified healthcare provider.

This book is intended as general information only, and should not be used to diagnose or treat any health condition. In light of the complex, individual, and specific nature of health problems, this book is not intended to replace professional medical advice. The ideas, procedures, and suggestions in this book are intended to supplement, not replace, the advice of a trained medical professional. Consult your physician before adopting any of the suggestions in this book, as well as about any condition that may require diagnosis or medical attention. The author and publisher disclaim any liability arising directly or indirectly from the use of this book.

Cover design by Frank Rivera.
Cover image © serezniy/123RF.

This book is available at quantity discounts for bulk purchases.
For information, please call 1-800-289-0963.

CONTENTS

PART 2: BEAUTY AND PERSONAL CARE   73

Chapter 3: Skin Care   74

Chapter 4: Hair and Body Care   96

Dedication

For my amazing husband, Jimmy, and our three beautiful children, Lilly, Lonni, and JD, who make every day better than the last!

Acknowledgments

I would like to take this opportunity to make special mention of the wonderful fathers I have been blessed to have in my life: my grandfather, Harry Allen, a wonderful man I look up to in so many ways, as a family man, teacher, coach, friend, and the father of my amazing Dad. My father, Brian Allen, who has been the most powerful influence in my life, showing me that it is possible to be strong, driven, and successful while also making life about the people you love, having fun, and making the most out of every day in life. My father-in-law, Steve Brandon, whose loving, creative, and fun personality not only makes him great company, but has also helped create the man of my dreams. And, my wonderful husband, Jimmy, who takes my breath away every day with his strength, support, and love that has surpassed everything I could ever hope for in a husband and a friend.

My amazing editors at Adams Media, Lisa Laing, Brendan O'Neill, and Jacqueline Musser: I thank you for giving me the opportunity to pursue my love of writing on topics about which I have such a strong passion.

I especially want to thank Skye Alexander for helping to edit this title with an amazing eye and technique that has surpassed anything and everything an author could hope for in a development editor; I consider this title a shared accomplishment achieved with the assistance of this amazing woman, whom I would have never met had it not been for this book.

INTRODUCTION

If you heard about an all-natural product that could prevent *and* treat illnesses, one that actually worked and had an outstanding track record, wouldn't you want to learn more about it? What if this was a tried-and-true remedy that has been widely used by cultures around the world for centuries and prized for its effectiveness in combating countless physical ailments? But wait, there's more. In addition to its many health benefits, this product can make you more beautiful by doing everything from whitening your teeth and stimulating hair growth to nixing acne and speeding weight loss. If this sounds too good to be true, I'm here to tell you that this product *does* exist—and it's available at every major supermarket and health food store. It might even be in your kitchen cupboard right now. What's this wondrous, magical elixir? It's coconut oil!

Modern medicine opts to treat and prevent every conceivable malady with pills, prescriptions, and procedures, but the recommended treatments, services, and medicines are often expensive, ineffective, or accompanied by undesirable or dangerous side effects. Although some medical breakthroughs are nothing short of miracles, we shouldn't rule out gentle, safe, effective natural healing products such as apple cider vinegar and—you guessed it—coconut oil. With its powerful antiviral, antibacterial, and antimicrobial properties, coconut oil can treat a host of health issues quickly, inexpensively, and without the risk of harmful side effects.

In this book, I show you how to use coconut oil to improve your life in 100 different ways. I've even included a number of healthy recipes and body-care products you can make yourself. Whether you're looking for a quick energy lift, a way to lose weight, or relief from eczema or athlete's foot, coconut oil can offer a solution. It can improve your sleep, digestion, and vitality as well. Coconut oil's health-boosting properties can safely treat internal and external issues by combating germs, bacteria, and viruses. By enhancing the quality of your life in numerous ways, coconut oil can let you live each and every day with less illness and stress. That's why I created this book: to show you an astounding number of easy and effective ways coconut oil can dramatically improve your life.

If you're ready to let coconut oil help you enjoy a healthier, happier, better life, then let's get started!

COCONUT OIL'S MANY HEALTH BENEFITS

Despite their name, coconuts aren't nuts. They're actually the fruit (scientifically termed *drupes*) that drops from the lovely palm fronds atop the beautiful coconut palms inhabiting tropical areas of the world. Named by sixteenth-century Spanish settlers, *coconut* derives from the Spanish word *coco*, used to refer to the skull. They coined the term because they thought the three indentations on the coconut's fibrous outer coating resembled a skull's two eyes and nose.

Originating in the tropical landscapes of Florida and the numerous tropical islands around the world, coconut palms provide us with a plentiful crop—55 million tons per year. Coconuts actually account for up to 60 percent of some Pacific cultures' diets. In economic trade, medicinal treatments, and nutrition, the coconut has established itself as one of the most important natural resources known to humankind.

The History of Coconut Oil

Coconut fossils dating back 55 million years have been discovered in parts of Australia and India, yet earlier fossils found in parts of the Americas lead some researchers to theorize that South America and southern North America may have been the coconut palm's birthplace. The coconut's ability to germinate even after the fruit has traveled the earth's oceans for 100 days or over 3,000 miles has made it difficult to determine where the coconut originated. Regardless of the coconut's birthplace, its importance in myriad cultures throughout time is evident in multiple written works dating back 1,500 years.

Although Pacific cultures had utilized coconut oil's medicinal powers for centuries, the Americas only learned of its healing properties in the mid-eighteenth century. Coconut oil's ability to combat bacteria, fungi, viruses, parasites, and microbes quickly made it a commodity of high demand in the Americas. In only a few decades after its introduction in the early 1900s, the oil's popularity skyrocketed. Finding the best method for extracting and processing the oil quickly became a focus for manufacturers worldwide.

Two methods were identified for developing coconut oil: "dry" and "wet." The dry process involved drying the "meat" of the coconut using heat, sunlight, or chemical solvents, followed by pressing the oil directly from the meat. The wet process compressed the coconut meat to expel the liquid and then separated the oil from the water via fermentation, boiling, or various chemical processes. Because the wet process required the use of heavy machinery, was more expensive, and often resulted in a lower yield, the dry process became the more common procedure used to produce coconut oil. Once the chemical solvents in the manufacturing process were replaced with natural treatment alternatives that were not exorbitantly expensive, the dry process became even more appealing to manufacturers. To this day it remains the go-to process for extracting and developing coconut oil.

The Unique Fat in Coconut Oil

Because of its high saturated-fat content, coconut oil was once thought to be unhealthy. However, researchers studying its unique properties stumbled upon an important difference between coconut oil and other high-saturated-fat foods. They discovered that coconut oil contains a unique type of saturated fat, classified as *lauric acid*, to which the body responds differently than it does to any other saturated fat.

Lauric Acid

Lauric acid is found in other natural sources, such as breastmilk. This twelve-carbon fatty acid is enzymatically digested, shuttled straight to the liver, and metabolized into a monoglyceride called *monolaurin*. During the digestive process, coconut oil's lauric acid increases energy levels and stamina, and boosts "good" cholesterol (HDL) levels. In addition, lauric acid and monolaurin act as antibacterial, antifungal, antiviral, and antimicrobial agents that potentially safeguard against common illnesses and ailments of the viral, bacterial, fungal, and microbial sort.

Different Types of Fatty Acids

Fatty acid chains of different lengths affect the body differently. Fats are classified in two ways:

1. By the type of saturation
2. By the length or size of the fatty-acid chain

"Saturation" is further broken down into different categories: saturated, monounsaturated, polyunsaturated, etc. The classification is used to describe the type and number of bonds that make up the fat molecule. The length of the fatty acid's "carbon chain" of carbon and hydrogen atoms is what determines a fat's classification as a short-chain fatty acid (SCFA), medium-chain fatty acid (MCFA), or long-chain fatty acid (LCFA). Long-chain fatty acids are found in animal and dairy products—they're the ones that can contribute to the buildup of plaque in arteries, increased LDL cholesterol, etc. Coconut oil is composed of medium-chain fatty acids or medium-chain triglycerides (MCTs), which help the body rather than harming it.

The Special Benefits of Coconut Oil

Okay, I realize you may be dubious about all these supposedly great things coconut oil can do for you. We've been taught to be skeptical of anything that sounds too good to be true—and for good reason. When medications promise to deliver outstanding results but also create sneaky side effects, when foods promise to be fat-free but are packed full of lots of unhealthy ingredients and calories, or when a new product assures us it can help us lose weight overnight with no effort at all, we know to be wary of the claims and skeptical about the results.

Coconut oil, however, is one of the few products where consumer skepticism is *not* warranted. Scientific research and peer-reviewed studies present evidence to demonstrate the amazing powers of coconut oil in improving virtually every area of your health . . . and your quality of life. For example:

- A study published in *Skin Pharmacology and Physiology* in 2010 determined that coconut oil had a beneficial effect in treating wounds.
- A study published in 2012 in the *Evidence-Based Complementary and Alternative Medicine Journal* discovered that coconut oil helped to prevent bone loss due to osteoporosis, and improved bone structure.
- A study published in *Neurobiology of Aging* in 2004 showed that medium-chain fatty acids improved memory recall in Alzheimer's patients.
- A study published in the *Journal of Cosmetic Science*'s March/April 2003 issue found that coconut oil conditioned and improved damaged hair, and protected hair from further damage.

And that's just the tip of the iceberg!

The main components responsible for providing all these different, effective benefits are medium-chain triglycerides (or "medium-chain fatty acids"), lauric acid, and capric acid. These multipurpose agents fight to prevent illness, improve immunity, and safeguard the health of your body externally and internally. Coconut oil's effectiveness is not just a gimmick or a fad.

One product and one simple lifestyle change can dramatically improve your overall well-being, providing benefits to your blood, metabolism functioning, digestion and nutrient absorption, and so much more. All you have to do is consume 1 to 3 tablespoons of coconut oil in its liquid or solid state daily to enhance your overall health and safeguard it for years to come.

You can store your coconut oil in your refrigerator or cabinet. When kept at a temperature higher than 75°F, coconut oil becomes liquid; at lower temperatures it solidifies. Either way, it provides the same benefits. The virgin, organic variety of coconut oil has a shelf life of fifteen months to three years, but I'm sure you'll use up your trusty container of coconut oil well before that length of time once you discover how many ways you can use it in your everyday life.

PART 1

HEALTH

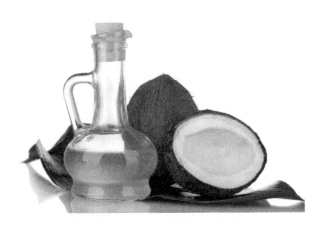

Chapter 1

NUTRITION

We all know that eating a balanced diet is essential to good health, and most of us realize that a healthy diet consists of plenty of fresh fruits and veggies, quality protein, and whole grains. Yet if you're like a lot of people, you don't always have the time or energy to plan and prepare meals that achieve your nutritional ideal. Our busy lifestyles have spawned a mammoth industry: dietary supplements. According to the National Institutes for Health, in 2012 people in the United States spent $32.5 billion on dietary supplements—and that doesn't include prescription medications taken for digestive complaints, cholesterol problems, diabetes, and other woes related to diet.

During the last half of the twentieth century, researchers began examining the effects of consuming coconut oil by studying populations whose diets contained lots of coconut and by doing animal and human testing. They discovered that coconut oil is chock-full of healthy properties that can aid digestion, facilitate weight loss, increase energy, support your immune system, and much, much more.

So before you hand over your hard-earned money for supplements that may or may not prove helpful—and could even be harmful—check out the amazing health benefits of coconut oil. This all-natural product is one of the easiest, least-expensive, and tastiest ways to improve your diet and your overall health.

1. SUPPLEMENT PRENATAL NUTRITION

Pregnancy makes additional demands on your body, so it's important to get ample amounts of essential nutrients to ensure that both mom and baby are receiving everything they need. Coconut oil can be a safe, all-natural addition to a pregnant woman's daily diet, providing astounding amounts of healthy saturated fat for her growing baby, her own dietary needs, and proper hormone production. In addition, the antiviral, antibacterial, and antimicrobial properties of the lauric acid in coconut oil (discussed earlier) help safeguard both mother and baby from illnesses before, during, and after pregnancy.

Because coconut oil boosts the immune system naturally, it can reduce the incidence of colds and flus commonly contracted during pregnancy.

> START WITH ½ TO 1 TABLESPOON OF COCONUT OIL PER DAY, AND GRADUALLY INCREASE THE ADULT DOSAGE TO 1 TO 3 TABLESPOONS PER DAY.

Drink your coconut oil neat, add it to your meals, or mix it into smoothies, juices, and teas to optimize your own health as well as your baby's.

By simply adding coconut oil to your daily diet, you can dramatically improve your diet's fat content, provide your body with a readily available fat source, and ensure that the quality of your fat intake is the healthiest possible.

ENSURE THE QUALITY OF YOUR COCONUT OIL

When purchasing coconut oil for optimal health benefits, choose organic, non-GMO, unrefined, and unpasteurized coconut oil. The minimal processing of the coconut oil will ensure that you receive the most nutrients and naturally occurring properties of coconut oil.

2. IMPROVE HORMONE PRODUCTION

Did you know that your hormone production is directly affected by your diet? Specifically, the amount and type of fats you consume directly influence the efficiency and productivity of your hormone-producing glands and organs. A number of glands are involved in the process of hormone production and regulation, including the pineal, thymus, thyroid, and pituitary glands. Your glands work closely with the pancreas to utilize the cholesterol and fats in the blood stream to produce the hormones that control the many processes constantly occurring in the body. When a disruption occurs because of a lack of these essential building blocks in amount or quality, hormonal problems result.

To make sure you're getting what you need, you can take the amounts of coconut oil recommended previously in "Supplement Prenatal Nutrition." Or, drink this delicious tropical fruit smoothie daily.

TO MAKE 1 CUP OF THIS PIÑA COLADA SMOOTHIE, COMBINE:

1 tablespoon coconut oil
1 cup pineapple
1 frozen banana

Place coconut oil into a high-speed blender. Add fruit. Blend on high speed until all ingredients are emulsified and well blended. Smoothie should be frothy and free of solid coconut oil bits.

HORMONE LEVELS AFFECT EVERYTHING

From the maintaining quality of your blood and brain functioning to improving or reducing your chances of conceiving, your hormone levels impact every single process that occurs in your body. With a quality diet of essential nutrients, you can ensure your hormone levels stay at optimum levels.

3. SOOTHE HEARTBURN

Heartburn is the burning sensation experienced when the stomach's digestive acids reflux into the esophagus. This uncomfortable condition is the consequence of the body's response to a disturbance of the necessary stomach acids produced to digest stomach contents. Heartburn can last from minutes to days and is readily treated with over-the-counter medications and antacids. Although these temporary pain relievers may help the discomfort in the moment, they do not treat the underlying issue. This is where coconut oil can help, naturally.

TO EASE HEARTBURN AND BALANCE STOMACH ACIDS, USE:

1 tablespoon coconut oil at the onset, then ¼ tablespoon every 30 minutes

Continue ingesting coconut oil until heartburn subsides.

Coconut oil is a "healthy fat" that supports the natural balance of digestive juices in the stomach, aids the body in maintaining proper digestion, quickly moves harmful elements (in foods and drinks) from the stomach, and normalizes the stomach acids' pH balance. It is one of the few fats that quickly and safely acts to correct heartburn by preventing a disruption in the normal process of digestion, restoring your stomach to normal.

CHARCOAL FOR HEARTBURN?

While searching through over-the-counter remedies for heartburn, you'll notice that charcoal is listed as the active ingredient in most medications. Although effective in combating heartburn, charcoal is a highly controversial ingredient and is strongly advised against for pregnant or nursing women.

4. CALM NAUSEA

Whether your nausea is a result of pregnancy, an undesirable aftereffect of your diet, or the unwanted side effect of an illness, the queasiness of nausea can be as uncomfortable and debilitating (sometimes more so) as actually vomiting.

A number of old wives' tales profess the effectiveness of formulas and techniques intended to calm nausea, but few have received attention for actually being helpful. One that's growing in popularity is coconut oil. With its calming, neutralizing capabilities that reverse the uncomfortable effects of stomach acid gone awry, coconut oil can help quell an upset stomach within minutes. Before turning to your local pharmacy or supermarket for over-the-counter medications that contain questionable ingredients or may cause side effects, try a couple of the following coconut oil combinations that could provide long-lasting relief in no time:

- Add 1 tablespoon coconut oil to a cup of stomach-soothing hot ginger tea.

- Toss ½ cup spinach leaves with 1 tablespoon coconut oil and ½ tablespoon apple cider vinegar, and eat.

- Consume ¼ to ½ tablespoon coconut oil, in its liquid or solid state.

By reducing the amount of processed foods and drinks in your diet and improving the quality of the whole foods you consume, you can avoid nausea and vomiting naturally by preventing it before it starts.

GINGER: THE STOMACH SOOTHER

When searching for the right ginger product to remedy your stomach issues, you may be tempted to reach for a cold glass of ginger ale. However, few commercial products these days contain natural ginger and therefore lack its beneficial properties. Opt instead for real gingerroot that you can eat, brew in teas, or cook in foods for maximum benefits and relief.

5. AID DIGESTION

Digestive issues are among the most prevalent problems plaguing people in the United States today. Due to the Standard American Diet (appropriately referred to by its acronym "SAD") consisting of calorie-dense, nutrient-deficient foods and drinks, many people suffer from digestive issues that range from indigestion and constipation to malabsorption of essential vitamins and minerals. If you fall into this category, fret not. Coconut oil is here to save the day! By consuming just ½ to 1 tablespoon of coconut oil before or with meals, you can help your body easily digest your food.

Medium-chain triglycerides (MCTs) are the digestive-system-saving elements that separate coconut oil from other fats found in foods that commonly cause disruption in the stomach's natural acid balance. When you consume MCTs, the entire process by which digestion occurs is different. MCTs are quickly broken down into medium-chain fatty acids (discussed earlier in this chapter), absorbed into the intestines, and transported directly to the liver for processing in a manner that's more similar to a carbohydrate for fuel than a fat for storage. In this way, coconut oil does not require the usual processing for fats that causes the digestive system, lymphatic system, and blood stream to work strenuously in the "breakdown" process. By helping the body to absorb nutrients and deal with fats easily, coconut oil (consumed before or during meals) reduces digestive issues and aids your body in processing essential elements in your food.

Additionally, you can improve your digestion by:

- Consuming a diet of whole, unprocessed foods free of preservatives
- Eating smaller meals more frequently throughout the day

This will maximize the absorption of your diet's nutrients and reduce the incidence of digestive complaints.

6. INCREASE NUTRIENT ABSORPTION

Nutritional deficiencies cause illnesses and diseases that wreak havoc on the world's population—and not only in poor nations. With proper nutrition, the body is able to function properly and fend off illnesses; therefore, a quality diet is a lifesaver, literally. Each bite of food you consume contains nutrients that serve as the building blocks your body needs to perform everyday functions: provide energy; digest food; and maintain the health of your brain, heart, organs, and bones.

Coconut oil increases the body's absorption of necessary vitamins and minerals—by as much as eighteen times—when you add it to foods or consume it prior to eating. Put a single tablespoon into your food, or take 1 tablespoon 1 to 3 times per day to ensure that your body can absorb and utilize the nutrients you need. As *New York Times* bestselling author Dr.

Joseph Mercola explained in his article about coconut oil "Which Oil Will Help You Absorb Nutrients Better?" on his website *www.mercola.com*, "not all oils are created equal when it comes to nutrient absorption. . . . Some work better than others and can actually enhance the amount of nutrients your body receives from the food you eat."

When your body is deficient in vitamins or minerals, it is forced to limit the processes in which those elements are used—it may even extract those essentials from the existing stores found in the blood, organs, and bones. Deficiencies make the body more susceptible to illnesses and diseases that it could fight off if it were healthy. By adding coconut oil to your daily diet, you'll improve the overall quality of your health and safeguard against possible illness.

7. REPLACE FRIED FISH WITH HEALTHY COCONUT-CRUSTED FISH

If you love the crispy, crunchy texture of fried fish, but avoid eating it because of the unhealthy fats and oils used in cooking it, this tasty dish using coconut oil will win you over. In many tropical regions of the world—especially those located on the ocean—cooking seafood in coconut oil is commonplace. For generations, the people of Hawaii, the Philippines, India, and coastal areas of Asia have enjoyed flavorful and healthful dishes that combine fresh fish with coconut oil, spices, and maybe a splash of lime. Although you can use any type of fish you prefer, this Coconut-Crusted Fish recipe is best suited to white fish such as haddock, cod, halibut, sea bass, or tilapia.

TO MAKE 4 SERVINGS OF THIS LIGHT AND FLAVORFUL COCONUT-CRUSTED FISH, COMBINE:

¼ cup coconut oil
½ teaspoon salt
4 (5-ounce) fish fillets

½ cup crushed nuts (pecans or macadamia nuts)
½ cup shredded, unsweetened coconut
2 tablespoons crushed panko bread crumbs
Olive oil to grease pan

Preheat oven to 400°F. Prepare a 9" × 13" pan, lightly coating the bottom and sides with olive oil.

Combine coconut oil and salt in a bowl; toss fish in mix to coat.

Combine nuts, coconut, and panko in a second bowl; turn fish in mixture to coat completely, and place into prepared pan.

Bake for 15 to 20 minutes, or until fish is cooked through.

Add mango salsa or serve atop peppery rice, and enjoy this flavorful fish with your favorite veggies.

8. SPEED WEIGHT LOSS

In order to effectively lose weight, three basic components must be present in your daily diet and routine:

1. Caloric deficit
2. Increased calorie burning
3. Essential nutrients required for efficient metabolic processing

Coconut oil can play an amazing role in any weight-loss program. It provides a clean, quality fat that improves calorie burn because it is processed differently than other fats. Its medium-chain fatty acids that are broken down easily for energy use not only help to improve your body's calorie burn and metabolic functioning, but also replace the traditional fats that often get stored in your body instead of used. Therefore, coconut oil improves your digestion, nutrient absorption, and energy levels. By consuming just 1 tablespoon of coconut oil 2 to 3 times daily, you can boost the benefits of your daily diet and easily speed weight loss.

One pound is equal to 3,500 calories, and you can expect to lose one pound of weight by creating a deficit of that amount.

- By cutting calories in the amount of 500 per day, or increasing physical activity by one walk, run, swim, or bike ride totaling a 500-calorie expenditure per day, you can expect to lose one pound per week.
- By improving your body's calorie-burning capabilities, you can further improve that weekly weight loss by eating six small meals instead of three larger ones. If you're consuming three daily meals that average 500 calories each for a total of 1,500 daily calories, you can improve your body's calorie-burning efficiency by consuming six 250-calorie meals instead.
- Finally, if you can improve the quality of the nutrients contained in those six daily meals by eating a diet based on whole, nutrient-dense foods and clean fats, you can further speed weight loss.

9. INCREASE FAT LOSS

People often have the misconception that the body burns fat in the same way that it burns calories. This notion could not be further from the truth! The body feeds on dietary fat, utilizing the fat it needs for energy and storing any excess as, well, fat. A deficiency of fat forces the body into hibernation mode, which sets into motion a fat-storing process. In order to speed fat loss, you have to make healthy or "clean" fats a readily available part of your daily diet. By doing this, your body does the exact opposite of the hibernation-mode fat storing and instead begins to burn those fats efficiently as fuel. What happens when your body becomes an efficient fat-burning machine? It turns to your fat stores for energy. This means that hard-to-lose fat quickly and efficiently gets used as fuel and (quite literally) disappears.

By eating whole, unprocessed foods such as fruits, vegetables, and lean meats, along with minimal grains and only clean fats (such as coconut and olive oils) and nuts, you can improve your fat-burning capabilities. To your clean diet, add a dose of 1 tablespoon of coconut oil by itself or in your food preparation 3 times per day. You'll soon transform your body into an efficient fat-burning machine.

THE BIG FAT LIE

Diet fads come and go, but one dangerous diet that somehow managed to survive decades of research pointing to the importance of fat in a healthy diet is the "low-fat" diet craze. We now know that diets low in fat can pose a host of health and lifestyle-inhibiting issues that actually prevent weight loss. These diets also contribute to a lack of energy and proper system functioning throughout the body and brain.

10. GAIN IMMEDIATE ENERGY

We have come to expect an "afternoon slump," a drop in energy in the latter part of the day. Although lack of sleep, irregular sleep patterns, and unhealthy lifestyle habits can adversely affect your energy levels, it is more likely that a poor diet lacking in quality nutrients is the energy-zapping culprit. When your body is deficient in any of the macronutrients (carbohydrates, proteins, and fats) or micronutrients (vitamins and minerals), it lacks the ability to produce the energy you need to perform well.

What's the best type of fuel you can provide to your body for immediate energy? Look no further than coconut oil. A study published in the *American Journal of Clinical Nutrition* found that coconut oil's medium-chain triglycerides improved energy expenditure. Digested easily, shuttled directly to the liver, and used as energy to burn, coconut oil is a clean, immediately available fuel that doesn't require lengthy digestive processing and breakdown.

WHEN YOU FEEL FATIGUED, USE:

1 tablespoon of coconut oil

Consume it any way you like to "perk up" quickly, without the crash that comes after ingesting sugar or caffeine.

Your body achieves its goal of reserving energy by limiting your energy output, and it does this by reducing the energy available. Becoming aware of this cause-and-effect situation can help you recognize your body's cues (tiredness or fatigue) for what they really are: a cry for help and the nutrients it can utilize as fuel. By adding 3 tablespoons per day of coconut oil to your diet, you can easily avoid that "afternoon slump" and stay sharp throughout the day.

11. ENJOY NUTRIENT-RICH SPINACH PESTO WITH COCONUT OIL

When you were a kid, did your mother insist that you "eat your spinach"? And remember those old Popeye cartoons that showed how eating spinach gave the sailor superhuman strength? Spinach is rich in iron, necessary for healthy blood, as well as vitamins A, B_2, C, K, and folic acid, plus manganese and magnesium. Its phytochemicals aid eyesight and provide anti-inflammatory and cancer-fighting benefits. Combine all these qualities with coconut oil's quality, medium-chain fatty acids and you've got a recipe for good health.

SERVED AS A DELICIOUS SPREAD ON BRUSCHETTA OR AS A SIMPLE DIPPING SAUCE FOR ROLLED MEATS AND CHEESES, THIS PESTO RECIPE MAKES AN OUTSTANDING APPETIZER FOR 6.

¼ cup pine nuts
3 cloves garlic, peeled
1½ cups basil leaves
1 cup spinach leaves
½ cup coconut oil
Salt and pepper to taste

In a small skillet over medium heat, slightly toast pine nuts until fragrant, about 2 to 5 minutes.

In a blender or food processor, combine pine nuts, garlic, basil, and spinach; blend or process on high while adding coconut oil gradually until desired consistency is achieved.

Season with salt and pepper to taste.

You can also add a good-sized dollop of this tasty pesto atop your favorite pasta dish to give it some extra zip, as well as additional nutrients.

12. IMPROVE CHOLESTEROL LEVELS

When people speak of "cholesterol" they usually mean the scientifically termed LDL (low-density lipoprotein) cholesterol. LDL is the type of cholesterol responsible for contributing to plaque deposits that build up in the walls of the arteries. The gradual hardening of this built-up plaque is the main contributing factor to the condition known as *atherosclerosis* that can lead to heart attacks and strokes. On the opposite end of the spectrum lies the so-called "good" cholesterol, HDL, also known as high-density lipoprotein. It aids in reducing the buildup of plaque within the arteries by breaking plaque away from arterial walls and carrying the bits back to the liver to be passed out of the body.

Coconut oil is packed full of medium-chain triglycerides that contribute to the HDL cholesterol levels of the blood and aid the body in ridding itself of LDL cholesterol naturally. Only 1 to 3 tablespoons of coconut oil per day, taken by the spoonful or in food, can help improve the HDL cholesterol levels, thereby effectively reducing the levels of LDL effortlessly.

COCONUT OIL AND HEART HEALTH

After reviewing data regarding coconut-eating groups of people, Hans Kaunitz, MD, and Conrado S. Dayrit, MD, found that the available population studies showed that dietary coconut oil does not lead to high serum cholesterol or high coronary heart disease mortality or morbidity. Islanders from the Philippines and Polynesia who had high levels of coconut oil consumption in their diets showed no evidence of harmful effects from the coconut oil they consumed on a daily basis. (See *www .coconutresearchcenter.org* for more medical studies and information.)

13. REGULATE INSULIN

A staggering 30 percent of the U.S. population suffers from type 1 or type 2 diabetes, and that number is on the rise with close to 2 million new diabetes diagnoses every year. You might be surprised to learn that coconut oil is a helpful dietary addition to the diabetic's diet. A study done in 2009 at the Garvan Institute of Medical Research in Australia found that a diet rich in coconut oil protected against insulin resistance. By ingesting just ½ to 1 tablespoon of coconut oil prior to meals and snacks, many diabetics find relief from their blood sugar fluctuations and resulting symptoms, allowing them to return to a healthy lifestyle free of pinpricks and medications.

Coconut oil's abundance of specialized saturated fats made of lauric acid provide preventative health-boosting benefits, and its medium-chain fatty acids improve blood health and slow the rate by which food is digested. These fats have remarkable effects on regulating blood sugar levels and reducing spikes, thereby helping diabetics to maintain stable blood sugar levels throughout the day. Coconut oil's illness-preventing properties also help to maintain overall health.

Although a number of pharmaceutical drugs are available to treat diabetes, many of these drugs have harmful (and sometimes deadly) side effects. By eating a diet that is low in sugar and refined carbohydrates, that combines the macronutrients (carbohydrates, protein, and fats) in every meal, and that includes minimal polyunsaturated fats, many people with diabetes have been able to treat their insulin-resistant diagnoses naturally.

14. BOOST METABOLISM FUNCTIONING

Have you ever tried to lose weight by cutting calories drastically, only to be disappointed to find that you weren't losing weight? Your mind was not playing tricks on you. Your body's metabolism is an intricate system that acts and reacts according to what you eat. What most people don't understand is that strict limitations put on your diet can mean strict limitations put on your weight loss. Your metabolism can most easily be compared to a wood-burning stove. When you feed your body nutrient-dense foods, its metabolism burns quickly and efficiently, firing bright and strong. A burning fire requires a steady, similarly sized load of good clean-burning wood in order to maintain stable heat. If you stop feeding wood into that fire, it will smolder. If you give the fire poor quality wood, it will smolder. But if you maintain that fire with a steady provision of the quality wood it needs, it will thrive.

Most natural fats, like those found in nuts, meat, and oils, will provide your body with what it needs to function throughout the day—but the specific fats in coconut oil surpass these others in giving your body what it needs to thrive. Coconut oil's medium-chain fatty acids require less energy to produce more energy than the long-chain fatty acids found in most foods laden with saturated fat—a thermogenic (heat-producing, metabolism-speeding) effect resulting from the digestion and processing of the coconut oil's lauric acid. Combined with coconut oil's blood-sugar stabilizing, craving-calming effects, you get a metabolism that burns fuel faster and more efficiently—just like a well-fed fire.

Take 1 tablespoon of coconut oil at least 3 times a day with food or prior to workouts. This ensures that your body has no reason to store fat but plenty of reason to burn it! In order to boost your metabolism even more, eat clean foods that are nutrient-dense, exercise every day (to keep your muscles growing and burning more calories, even at rest), and feed your body the necessary amount of healthy fats it needs to burn efficiently.

15. ENCOURAGE SATIETY

Have you ever felt that you were following a diet, giving your body what it needed with quality nutrition, and yet somehow your hunger wouldn't go away? If your caloric intake is adequate—and your daily activities aren't forcing your body to require more calories (thus the hunger cues)—you may wonder why you don't feel full and satisfied. Coconut oil can promote satiety, especially if you combine it with chia seeds. This good-for-you combination provides quality nutrition in a long-lasting, hunger-calming, energy-boosting substance that will transform your diet and exercise world.

COMBINE:

1 tablespoon coconut oil
½ tablespoon chia seeds

Allow the mixture to set for about 5 minutes. Consume the mixture on its own, in a drink, or in a meal.

Do this daily—or as often as you like—to benefit from the hours of satisfaction and improved energy that will follow. The gel-like substance that forms when chia seeds are mixed with a liquid (such as coconut oil) moves slowly through the digestive system, providing a stable amount of energy that continues to be available for many hours after ingestion.

Edible chia seeds derive from the desert plant *Salvia hispanica* and contain omega-3 fatty acids, carbohydrates, protein, fiber, antioxidants, and calcium. In the Mayan language, "chia" is derived from a word meaning strength. Aztec runners used chia seeds as a provision that helped them run hundreds of miles over a period of only a few days. The added benefit of this unique combination is a hunger-calming effect that results from the healthy fat being processed in the body while the slow-moving gel continues to signal the brain that the stomach is full and satisfied. Energy production stays high, as does your level of satisfaction.

16. SUBSTITUTE COCONUT OIL FOR EGGS IN RECIPES

Many recipes call for eggs as a binding agent. However, coconut oil can be used as a delicious, nutritious, vegan substitute. By using coconut oil as a binding agent in your culinary creations, you can produce the tasty treats you love with a product that improves and safeguards health.

Like an egg or egg white, coconut oil can be used wet or solidified. In your recipes, you can utilize this quality to advantage by combining it with your favorite ingredients in small amounts in place of an egg. Substituting 1 tablespoon of coconut oil for one egg is the most widely used method, but you can adjust this depending upon how much or how little you see the recipe needs. By adding the coconut oil in ¼ tablespoon increments, you can gauge how much of the oil is required to develop a smooth consistency that isn't runny.

THIS RECIPE FOR VEGAN COCONUT MACAROONS MAKES 2 DOZEN MOUTHWATERING COOKIES.

1 cup coconut sugar

½ cup coconut milk

2 tablespoons maple syrup

2 teaspoons vanilla extract

1 teaspoon sea salt

3 cups shredded, unsweetened coconut

½ cup coconut flour

Coconut oil to grease pan

Preheat oven to 350°F. Line a baking sheet with parchment paper.

In a medium-sized mixing bowl, combine coconut sugar, coconut milk, maple syrup, vanilla, and salt. Add shredded coconut and coconut flour; mix well.

Using a basting brush, lightly grease the parchment-lined baking sheet with coconut oil.

Form the mixture into 1-inch balls; place on parchment-lined baking sheet about 1 inch apart. Bake for 10 minutes, or until edges are golden brown.

After eating a few of these coconut-rich, egg-free cookies, you may never go back to your old recipe.

17. SUBSTITUTE COCONUT OIL FOR BUTTER

People who choose to eliminate dairy products from their diets, either for health or philosophical reasons, will love coconut oil as a dairy-free alternative. Although most people consider butter to be an oil, it is actually a dairy product created with a specialized process that churns cow's milk into a solidified state. If you're vegan or you're one of the many people who experience digestion problems or increased phlegm production when you eat dairy products, you can still enjoy your favorite foods by replacing butter with a delicious, health-boosting fat: coconut oil.

Slathered on toast or mixed into your favorite recipe, coconut oil not only tastes great, but also offers countless benefits without causing the adverse reactions that often follow dairy-product consumption. Not only does coconut oil deliver a similar "buttery" taste, it provides an impressive number of health benefits that you won't find in butter or margarine. Its medium-chain fatty acids contribute to improved digestion and increased metabolism, while its lauric acid provides illness-preventing properties against viruses, bacteria, and microbes. Simply use a similar amount of coconut oil in place of butter and you'll not only taste a delicious difference, you'll *feel* a difference, too.

THE "LOW-FAT," "NO-FAT" TRADEOFF

Decades ago, manufacturers began catering to a new hype that condemned fats as the culprit in weight gain. Companies began producing foods with "low-fat" or "fat-free" ingredients. These foods were sometimes packed with unhealthy ingredients such as MSG (monosodium glutamate) to maintain the texture and taste consumers wanted. But due to the loss of fat, these foods presented new health issues. MSG tricks the brain into feeling hungry or unsatisfied—even after you've consumed a large amount of food. The ingredient is also connected with a host of issues that adversely affect everything from the respiratory system to the neurological development in children.

18. USE IN HIGH-TEMPERATURE COOKING

When people refer to "high-temperature cooking," they're speaking of the specific cooking methods that require a higher heat than is normally used in our everyday cooking style. Stir-frying is one of the best-known high-temperature cooking methods. It requires a heat in excess of 350°F. For this type of cooking, you would normally use a vegetable oil because of its high smoke point and its tendency to not oxidize at high temperatures, as happens with olive oil. However, studies such as one published in 2013 in the *International Journal of Cancer* indicate that trans fatty acids in hydrogenated oils (such as vegetable oils, corn oils, and soybean oils) may pose cancer risks—so it's no surprise that stir-fry lovers have sought out a healthy oil alternative. They found everything they needed (and more) in coconut oil. Try this stir-fry recipe and enjoy delicious taste with added health benefits galore.

TO MAKE 4 SERVINGS OF THIS VIBRANT COCONUT CHICKEN STIR-FRY, COMBINE:

½ cup plus 2 tablespoons coconut oil, separated

4 large skinless, boneless chicken breasts, cut into bite-sized pieces

¼ cup water

2 large carrots, chopped

1 large yellow onion, chopped

1 cup sugar snap peas

4 garlic cloves, peeled and minced

¼ cup soy sauce

Prepare a large skillet or wok over medium-high heat with ½ cup coconut oil. Heat for 1 to 3 minutes or until fragrant.

Add chicken to the pan and stir until cooked through, removing any juices that remain.

Add water, vegetables, garlic, and soy sauce to chicken and stir until carrots and onions are cooked through, about 7 minutes.

Remove from heat and drizzle with remaining 2 tablespoons coconut oil; serve immediately alone or with steamed rice.

19. SUBSTITUTE FOR OTHER OILS IN BAKING

Baked goods usually contain lots of butter and unhealthy oils. If you like to bake, you can substitute coconut oil to create the delicious baked goods you love. At temperatures over 75°F, coconut oil turns from a solid to a liquid similar in texture to melted butter or vegetable oil, and can be substituted for those ingredients in baking recipes. In its solidified form, coconut oil can be used in the same ways as shortening or hardened butter. Try this twist on a favorite tropical dessert.

TO MAKE THIS BEAUTIFUL PINEAPPLE UPSIDE-DOWN CAKE THAT SERVES 12, COMBINE:

½ cup plus 3 tablespoons coconut oil, separated
1 cup light brown sugar
1 (20-ounce) can sliced pineapple
20 maraschino cherries
1 cup cake flour, sifted
1 teaspoon baking powder
¼ teaspoon salt
2 eggs
1 cup white sugar

Preheat oven to 350°F.

In a 10-inch cast-iron skillet over low heat, heat ½ cup of coconut oil. Remove from heat and sprinkle in brown sugar to coat the bottom of pan. Arrange pineapple slices to cover the bottom of the skillet, placing one cherry in the center of each pineapple slice and around them.

Stir together flour, baking powder, and salt in a mixing bowl.

Separate egg yolks from egg whites; beat egg whites and 2 tablespoons of coconut oil, adding sugar gradually and beating to form stiff peaks after each addition.

Beat egg yolks separately until thickened, and fold yolks and flour mixture into egg whites in an over-under motion.

Fold in the last tablespoon of coconut oil until well blended, and pour batter into the cast-iron skillet, evenly covering the pineapple slices.

Bake for 30 to 45 minutes, or until a toothpick inserted in the center comes out clean.

Loosen the edges of the cake with a butter knife and let cool for 5 minutes before inverting onto a serving plate.

20. SUBSTITUTE FOR OTHER OILS IN COOKING

Coconut oil provides a perfect alternative to butter or other cooking oils in casseroles, soups and stews, and pasta or rice dishes. You can enjoy the delicious flavors of your favorite dishes, while also adding the health benefits of coconut oil. In some cases, you might find that you and your family actually prefer the distinctive taste of coconut oil to what you ordinarily use. Try this delicious and nutritious curry recipe— you'll become an instant convert.

TO MAKE 8 SERVINGS OF THIS HEARTY COCONUT CURRY VEGETABLE SOUP, COMBINE:

1 cup coconut oil

1 cup yellow onion, chopped

3 yellow potatoes, cubed into ¼-inch chunks

1 cup celery, chopped

1 cup carrots, chopped

3 cloves garlic, minced

2 tablespoons curry powder

4 cups vegetable stock

Salt and pepper to taste

In a large pot over medium heat, heat 1 cup of coconut oil for 5 minutes; add onions, potatoes, celery, carrots, and garlic.

Stir vegetables, allowing them to sweat for about 10 minutes or until onions and celery are translucent.

Add curry to vegetables and stir for 2 to 3 minutes, or until curry and coconut oil form a paste-like consistency over the vegetables.

Add vegetable stock to the pot and bring to a boil.

Reduce heat to low. Cover and simmer for 30 to 45 minutes, or until vegetables are tender.

Remove from heat; add salt and pepper to taste.

HYDROGENATED OILS

Hydrogenated oils can wreak havoc on your digestive system, brain functioning, and the body's processes that require fat. Hydrogenated oils are often hidden in the most surprising of foods (crackers, cookies, cakes, and even powdered versions of spices). Look for hydrogenated oils— sometimes listed as trans fats—on the ingredient list so you can avoid them.

21. ADD FLAIR TO YOUR COFFEE

Coffee lovers have one thing in common: They look forward to their morning cup of joe as the perfect way to start their day. Without coffee, many people find it difficult to get going in the morning, let alone in the right direction. Coffee provides caffeine and specific phytonutrients such as powerful antioxidants, making it one of the healthiest and beneficial drinks to add to your diet, in moderation. But when you heap in spoonfuls of sugar, generous amounts of cream or milk, or unnatural sugary creamer additions, this antioxidant-rich brew becomes less than the healthy dietary staple it is on its own.

What would you say if I told you that there is an ingredient you can blend into your morning coffee to flavor, sweeten, and lighten your brew as effectively as a sugary creamer? What if I also told you this simple addition provides you with special fatty acids that help improve your energy, blood health, and fat-burning processes, while also stabilizing your blood sugar to reduce the chance of a caffeine "crash"?

TO MAKE THIS MIRACULOUS MORNING COFFEE ADDITIVE, USE:

1 teaspoon to 1 tablespoon coconut oil
1 cup of your favorite coffee or espresso

Blend on high speed for 30 to 60 seconds to turn your black coffee into a frothy, rich, creamy cup of java that hints at the tropics and gives your brain and body an instant, delightfully unexpected kick.

Coconut oil also happens to be the perfect pairing for tea—use it to jumpstart your morning or as a pick-me-up when your energy starts to flag in the afternoon.

SUGARY COFFEE ADDITIONS

When you add that sweetened coffee creamer to your morning cup of joe, keep an eye on the amount you use and double-check the nutrition facts to ensure you're not overloading your daily diet with sugar simply by enjoying a delicious cup of coffee.

Chapter 2

TOTAL WELLNESS

The World Health Organization summed it up nicely when it described health as "a state of complete physical, mental and social well-being, and not merely the absence of disease or infirmity." Every day we deal with health issues that plague both the body and the mind, preventing us from achieving the goal of total wellness. You probably know that eating a healthy diet, exercising regularly, and making other positive lifestyle changes can help to safeguard your health and prevent or correct many illnesses by strengthening your immune system. But you may not yet realize what an important contribution coconut oil can make to your overall well-being. This chapter will open your eyes to some of the numerous health benefits this all-natural, gentle, and effective product can bring you.

Whether you want to avoid contracting a cold or the flu, to prevent urinary tract and yeast infections, or to combat anxiety and depression, coconut oil can help. Its medium-chain fatty acids can improve everything from brain fog to blood circulation, while also supporting the body's major systems so they work optimally and synergistically. By simply adding coconut oil to your daily diet, you may be able to avoid those "new and improved" prescription and over-the-counter medications that promise solutions for every issue imaginable—and also avoid any harmful side effects. In this chapter, you'll learn more about the amazing benefits of coconut oil and find more than thirty ways to use the oil to achieve the level of health you've been seeking. If you're ready to breathe easy (literally) and start living healthier, read on!

22. ALLEVIATE ALLERGY SYMPTOMS

Anyone who suffers from allergies can tell you that every season brings a new set of challenges, and with every fluctuation in the weather comes the possibility of an allergy flare-up. Headaches, itchy eyes, sneezing, coughing, and more severe reactions such as sinus and respiratory infections make daily life more difficult. Pharmaceutical companies provide a wide range of treatment options that can help to resolve symptoms, but often these come with side effects such as drowsiness or jitters.

Allergy sufferers, look no further for a natural, safe, and effective way to ease symptoms—without unpleasant side effects. Add coconut oil to your daily diet to reduce the pain and discomfort allergies can cause.

AS AN INTERNAL AID, USE:

1 to 3 tablespoons of coconut oil

Ingest every day, alone or in food, to help prevent and diminish allergy symptoms. The oil's naturally occurring lauric acid works internally to strengthen the body's immune system and reduce reaction to allergens—seasonal or otherwise.

Coconut oil's antiviral, antibacterial, and antimicrobial properties can also help decrease your sensitivity to allergens and allergy conditions. Plus the anti-inflammatory and antihistamine properties inherent in the lauric acid, produced by coconut oil's medium-chain fatty acids, also help to relieve allergy symptoms such as sinus pressure, sneezing, and respiratory discomfort.

AS A TOPICAL PREVENTATIVE, USE:

A small amount of coconut oil

Dab oil on the inside of your nostrils to keep allergens from taking effect.

A number of other simple practices can help you stave off allergy reactions, naturally:

- Shower as soon as you come indoors to remove pollen and other allergens that may cling to your skin and hair.
- Drive with your windows closed, especially when pollen, ragweed, etc., counts are high.
- Eat local honey to build up your immunity to allergens in your area.

23. SHARPEN MENTAL CLARITY

You probably know that caffeine acts to boost mental clarity, but you may not know that coconut oil is also effective in improving mental alertness—quickly, naturally, and for longer durations than caffeine. When you consider that 60 percent of your brain is fat, it seems logical that feeding it a healthy fat—coconut oil—would make your gray matter function better. And, indeed, it does. Whether you're feeling sluggish in the morning, out of energy in the afternoon, or simply find yourself slipping into a "brain fog" at any time of the day, coconut oil can help. By adding 1 to 3 tablespoons of coconut oil to your daily diet, you can dramatically improve your mental alertness and maintain a higher level of cognitive functioning throughout the day. You can also add a dollop of coconut oil to your coffee or tea for a quick "pick me up" (see "Add Flair to Your Coffee" in Chapter 1.)

With medium-chain fatty acids that are quickly and easily digested, coconut oil has special stimulating effects on brain functioning that no saturated fat provides. Ingesting coconut oil provides immediate and long-lasting energy. This sudden stimulation "wakes up" your brain and improves your mental awareness and cognitive functioning, as discussed in "Gain Immediate Energy" in Chapter 1.

Studies have also shown that ingesting coconut oil significantly increases the production (and resulting number) of ketone bodies in the blood. Your brain requires "food" for energy and utilizes ketones for optimum nourishment. A 2013 study published in *Biomedical Journal* found the medium-chain triglycerides in a ketone-boosting diet to be "one of the most effective therapies for drug-resistant epilepsy." Coconut oil may even reduce the incidence of serious degenerative mental conditions such as Alzheimer's.

24. IMPROVE BLOOD CIRCULATION

Blood circulation affects everything from your mental functioning and energy level to your internal body temperature. If you experience bouts of fatigue, brain fog, or chilliness much of the time, poor circulation may be the culprit. The great news for anyone struggling with poor circulation is that coconut oil can easily and naturally improve your blood flow and stop those undesirable side effects within a matter of days.

Coconut oil's benefits to blood circulation begin when the liver minimally processes the oil and immediately makes it available to the blood. Once released into the blood, coconut oil's medium-chain fatty acids bind with "bad" cholesterol (LDL) and help to safely remove it from the blood stream, while simultaneously boosting the levels of good cholesterol (HDL). As a result, blood quality improves, metabolism rate increases, and the blood's circulation becomes more efficient.

TO OPTIMIZE YOUR CHOLESTEROL LEVELS AND RETURN YOUR CIRCULATION TO NORMAL, USE:

½ to 1 tablespoon of coconut oil

Ingest 3 times a day at regular intervals (most commonly, every six hours) for a total of up to 3 tablespoons daily. Take it neat by the spoonful, or add to your food.

In addition to the discomforts associated with poor blood circulation, dangerous outcomes can result from its effects on blood pressure, including cardiovascular disease, strokes, heart attacks, and other illnesses that result from circulatory malfunctions. You can take control of your circulation issues by becoming proactive in various other ways, too:

- Eat a proper diet.
- Exercise regularly.
- Make sure you get enough restful sleep.

25. EAT SWEET POTATOES WITH COCONUT TO BENEFIT YOUR BLOOD

Packed with beta-carotene, sweet potatoes can increase the amount of vitamin A in your blood. They're also rich in vitamin C, as well as a number of other vitamins and minerals. Although we usually think of sweet potatoes as being orange in color, there's a purple variety that contains lots of antioxidants, too. And this root veggie's dietary fiber can aid blood sugar regulation. This recipe combines the benefits of sweet potatoes with coconut oil's blood-strengthening lauric acid and ginger's digestive properties and makes a delicious, nutritious side dish for 8 diners.

TO SERVE THIS GINGER–SWEET POTATO CASSEROLE WITH COCONUT AS AN ACCOMPANIMENT TO YOUR HOLIDAY MEALS—OR ANYTIME, USE:

Coconut oil as needed to grease pan, plus 2 tablespoons
1 (13.5-ounce) can coconut milk
½ cup raw coconut sugar
1 tablespoon orange zest
½ teaspoon sea salt
3 inches fresh ginger, grated
½ teaspoon powdered nutmeg
⅛ teaspoon cloves

½ cup fresh coconut, grated, divided
4 cups sweet potatoes, thinly sliced

Preheat oven to 325°F. Grease a 9" × 9" baking pan with coconut oil until well coated.

In a small bowl, mix coconut milk, sugar, orange zest, salt, ginger, and spices.

In a small saucepan, melt 2 tablespoons coconut oil.

Mix ¼ cup coconut with sweet potatoes; add to the baking dish. Drizzle with warmed coconut oil, making sure sweet potatoes are well coated. Pour coconut milk mixture over sweet potatoes; stir until well mixed.

Bake, uncovered, for 30 minutes. Remove from oven and stir, paying close attention to the edges. Sprinkle with remaining fresh coconut and return to the oven. Bake for another 45 minutes. Remove from oven, and serve.

After you've tasted this healthier and zestier sweet potato dish, you'll never again make the old holiday standby topped with marshmallows.

26. REDUCE CONSTIPATION

Constipation is a common condition experienced by an astounding number of people each and every day. Like many other symptoms, constipation can be the result of a number of conditions from pregnancy or poor diet, or a side effect of taking medications or undergoing treatments for health problems. This uncomfortable situation can quickly turn from slightly painful to quite serious. Because everyone's "regularity"— the duration of time between regular bowel movements—can differ as much as hours or even days, it can be difficult to determine whether or not someone is battling constipation.

If you find yourself dealing with any of the following symptoms, you may be experiencing constipation:

- Feeling the urge to poop, to no avail
- Maximum effort yields minimal results
- Passing a bowel movement less than three times per week
- Stomach pain
- Incomplete bowel movements

The good thing about treating constipation early is that you can quickly and easily prevent the problem from worsening, alleviating the condition almost immediately. By addressing constipation with coconut oil, you can naturally reduce the uncomfortable situation and its resulting symptoms gradually.

1. Start by consuming 1½ tablespoons of coconut oil daily, in a solid or liquid state.
2. Refrain from eating any additional solids until the blockage is passed.
3. Consume an additional ½ tablespoon of coconut oil every half-hour over the course of four hours; only attempt to poop when the urge arises.

Whether the constipation is due to a buildup of unhealthy, nutrient-void foods, or a condition resulting from an infection, coconut oil's fast-acting lauric acid and capric acid help to move things along (literally) by assisting the digestive system and maintaining a healthy digestive tract free of constipation-causing health issues. If your constipation persists, contact a physician in order to rule out possible contributing conditions.

27. HELP HEAL HEMORRHOIDS

Hemorrhoids can produce anything from slight discomfort to excruciating pain. According to the Mayo Clinic, about 50 percent of people over the age of fifty suffer to some degree from hemorrhoids. Not only can coconut oil ease the unpleasantness of this common condition, it can also help prevent hemorrhoids from developing.

Hemorrhoids occur when a person pushes excessively while trying to pass a bowel movement—a situation that often results from poor digestion. When you consume a diet that is high in processed foods and "bad" fats (long-chain triglycerides such as those in corn oil, vegetable oils, and trans fats), low in fiber (found in fruits and vegetables), or high in sugar, the result can be a disastrous digestive issue that creates hard stools that can be difficult and painful to pass. Add 1 to 3 tablespoons of coconut oil to your daily diet and you'll soon notice improvement in your stool consistency and less frequency of hemorrhoids.

Coconut oil's medium-chain fatty acids and lauric acid minimize the frequency of hemorrhoids by improving digestion, promoting a healthy metabolism, and ensuring proper nutrient absorption. Coconut oil's antibacterial properties also fight off possible digestive "bugs," including viruses and bacteria that can impair proper digestive functioning. But the benefits don't stop there. If you use coconut oil topically to soothe hemorrhoids, you can reduce inflammation in the area, while combatting bacteria and germs and preventing the possibility of infection.

Also consider consuming a diet rich in whole, natural foods and make sure you drink at least 64 ounces of water per day (that is, one 8-ounce cup per hour over a period of eight hours) to help keep stools loose.

28. EASE IBS

Irritable Bowel Syndrome, also referred to as IBS, is a condition that causes bouts of inflammation in the colon. Not actually a disease, like Irritable Bowel Disease (IBD), IBS has two well-known, common conditions referred to as either "nervous colitis" or "spastic colon." Because IBS issues are not as chronic or severe as IBD conditions, the symptoms can be treated and prevented more easily.

TO PREVENT AND REDUCE THE INFLAMMA- TION CONNECTED WITH IBS, USE:

1 tablespoon of coconut oil

Ingest 1 to 3 times per day, either by itself or mixed into foods and drinks, to deter or ease IBS.

Coconut oil is a healthy form of fat that minimizes the work the digestive system has to do to break down the fat into lauric acid. Lauric acid, as discussed in Chapter 1, acts as an antimicrobial agent, safeguarding health and improving immunity. Coconut oil can help prevent the onset of IBS while also providing symptom relief once IBS develops.

Improving your lifestyle and diet can also help to alleviate IBS issues:

- Eat a diet focused on whole foods that provide an abundance of fiber.
- Drink at least 64 ounces of water per day.
- Minimize consumption of alcohol.
- Refrain from smoking.
- Limit the amount of sugar, unhealthy fat, and acidic foods in your daily diet.

29. CALM COLITIS AND CROHN'S SYMPTOMS

Irritable bowel disease, also known as IBD, is the term used to refer to the digestive issues that cause chronic inflammation and pain in the gut. Crohn's disease and colitis are two of the most common subsets of diseases that fall into the category of IBD. When healthy white blood cells attack the lining of the colon, mistakenly identifying a foreign or harmful "invader," Crohn's and colitis develop. The series of excruciating painful and debilitating symptoms are a direct result of the inflammation occurring within the stomach lining.

Although the two conditions fall within the same category of IBD, the differences between the two are significant. With Crohn's, the inflammation is not limited to just the gastrointestinal tract, and it can produce symptoms that range from nausea, abdominal pain, fever, and diarrhea to negative effects on the skin, eyes, joints, and liver. The severity of Crohn's can vary from individual to individual, but it commonly produces ulcers and blockages within the intestines, resulting from the chronic inflammation and swelling. Colitis,

while also severe, is more commonly contained within the colon and is a result of germ-resistance issues. White blood cells attack the food and bacteria in the stomach, and produce symptoms that include fatigue, loss of appetite, bloody stools, and anemia. Coconut oil's soothing consistency and remarkable anti-inflammatory properties aid the digestive system and gastrointestinal tract.

TO EASE IBD CONDITIONS, USE:

1 to 3 tablespoons of coconut oil

Ingest each day, either neat or in your food. The oil's antibacterial, antimicrobial, and antiviral properties can provide relief from illnesses that can agitate and compound the symptoms of IBD issues.

At present, there is no cure for IBD. However, coconut oil can promote proper digestion, calm ulcers, improve bowel consistency, and maintain a quality of health within the gastrointestinal system that IBD sufferers will welcome.

30. PREVENT COLDS AND RESPIRATORY INFECTIONS

Respiratory conditions can range in severity from a common cough to pneumonia and can cause mild to major discomfort. Bacterial and viral infections are all around us, all the time, and can quickly take advantage of a weakened immune system and grow into a full-blown illness. If you feel tightness in your chest or a "rattle" in your lungs when you breathe, you may think that a cold has taken hold and there's nothing you can do. But you'd be wrong!

inflammation of the lungs and sinuses. Ingesting a dose of 1 tablespoon a day can minimize discomfort and shorten the duration of your illness. Although many people turn to extra doses of vitamin C or over-the-counter medications that promise to provide cold prevention in the winter months—the "flu season"—you may want to consider adding coconut oil to your overall wellness program all year long.

TO BOOST YOUR IMMUNITY, USE:

1 to 3 tablespoons of coconut oil

Ingest daily, by itself or in your food. Providing powerful lauric acid and capric acid that directly combat bacteria, viruses, and other harmful infections that can attack your respiratory system, coconut oil makes for the perfect prevention and solution.

Once you've come down with a cold, coconut oil's illness-fighting properties can bring relief by reducing

THE GREAT DAIRY DEBATE

For years, the "dairy debate" has tried to determine whether dairy products contribute to respiratory conditions. It's well known that eating dairy products produces phlegm—but are milk and other dairy products culprits in a number of respiratory issues? Even if you aren't lactose intolerant, you may opt to eliminate dairy products from your diet.

31. REDUCE THE DURATION/SEVERITY OF THE FLU

The flu is one of the most well-known and feared illnesses. Infecting millions of people of all ages every year, the flu has gained notoriety because of its long-lasting, severe symptoms that can cause everything from fever and chills to death. Since 1976, the average number of deaths in the United States from the flu ranged from 3,000 to 49,000—numbers high enough to warrant major concern, especially among individuals who may be exposed to environments and/or people with the flu virus. Coconut oil offers an effective, all-natural alternative for the prevention, treatment, and recovery from the flu.

TO COMBAT THE FLU QUICKLY, SAFELY, AND EFFECTIVELY, USE:

1 to 3 tablespoons of coconut oil

Take daily, in food or in liquid form.

Coconut oil's medium-chain fatty acids naturally produce antibacterial, antiviral, antifungal, and antimicrobial properties within the body. These provide protection against the flu by strengthening your immune system and helping it to fend off illnesses. Coconut oil's antiviral properties can also help to rid the body of the flu virus and reduce the duration and severity of the flu if you do contract it.

Flu vaccines provide about a 74-percent reduction of flu infection (in persons over the age of six months), but they may cause adverse reactions, even illness. A number of over-the-counter remedies also claim to prevent the flu, minimize the duration and severity of the illness, or relieve symptoms associated with the virus; however, these medications are created with questionable ingredients that can lead to unwanted side effects. Instead, play it safe and use coconut oil instead.

CAN COCONUT OIL KILL VIRUSES?

In 1966, Dr. Jon Kabara figured out that certain medium-chain fatty acids (lauric acids) in coconut oil actually kill some viruses. Dr. Kabara said, "Never before in the history of man is it so important to emphasize the value of lauric oils." The medium-chain fats and monoglycerin in coconut oil are similar to fats in mothers' milk and have similar nutraceutical effects.

32. SOOTHE A SORE THROAT

If you've ever suffered from a sore throat you know that the condition can not only be painful, it can also interfere with your daily life. Normal sleep patterns get interrupted. You can't eat your regular diet due to difficulty swallowing. Even communication becomes limited because of the strain speaking causes. A sore throat can seem a minor illness, but why suffer from it if you don't have to?

When you consume a tablespoon of coconut oil, its illness-fighting properties get to work immediately. By coating the inside of the throat, the oil begins the healing process, and its anti-inflammatory properties help alleviate the discomfort. By ingesting 1 to 3 tablespoons of coconut oil per day, you can improve your immunity and help safeguard your health against illnesses that cause sore throats.

Coconut oil's lauric acid acts as an antibacterial, antiviral, antimicrobial agent, helping to rid the body of infection and eliminate the source of the sore throat. Even antibiotic-resistant strains of viruses often respond well to coconut oil, making coconut oil one of the most effective natural pain relievers available. It not only minimizes the amount of discomfort you experience, it also shortens the length of time you suffer with a sore throat and reduces the chance of the recurring illnesses that commonly cause a sore throat.

APPLE CIDER VINEGAR FOR SORE THROATS

Gargling with a combination of 1 teaspoon apple cider vinegar and 1 tablespoon warm water provides antibacterial, antiviral, and antimicrobial properties that can help fend off the cause of a sore throat. Add this daily practice to your coconut oil regimen to help restore the throat's natural health.

33. RELIEVE DEPRESSION

According to *www.healthline.com/health/depression*, 10 percent of people in the United States suffer with depression—and that number is increasing. A number of contributing factors such as financial worries, family problems, job stress, or your environment can combine to create depression. Although genetic inheritance plays a part in the severity and frequency of bouts of depression, you can minimize your depression experiences or even eliminate them altogether. First, acknowledge that you are in control of your life and how you feel about your life and yourself. Then you can better grasp the simple steps you can take to help alleviate your depression and its symptoms.

1. Add coconut oil to your daily diet in the amount of 1 to 3 tablespoons. Your body and brain will benefit from the powerful immunity-promoting, cleansing, and health-improving properties for which the oil has become recognized.
2. Identify the areas of your life that you feel need improvement and commit to making the changes necessary to improve those areas.
3. Outline the steps needed to improve those areas. Set goals that will help you make those improvements, to achieve the life you want to have, and become the person you want to be.
4. Implement the necessary changes that will improve those areas of your life.
5. Eat and drink to live! Nourish your body and brain with coconut oil, nutrient-rich foods, and pure water. These dietary changes will have a profound impact on how you look and feel, while minimizing fluctuations in your energy level, mental clarity, cognition, and mood.

TAKE NIACIN TO ALLEVIATE DEPRESSION

From Bill W., the founder of Alcoholics Anonymous, comes a well-documented case for treating depression with niacin. He self-prescribed niacin (a B vitamin commonly deficient in people struggling with depression) to improve his own depression. Not only was Bill W. able to effectively treat his depression for the rest of his life with a daily dose of niacin, he also alleviated his issues with alcohol, as a result of the niacin easing his depression.

34. ALLEVIATE ANXIETY

What causes anxiety? There are as many answers to this question as there are people—and according to the Anxiety and Depression Association of America's Facts & Statistics, "Anxiety disorders are the most common mental illness in the U.S., affecting 40 million adults in the United States age 18 and older (18 percent of U.S. population)." (See *www.adaa.org/about-adaa/press-room/facts-statistics* for more information.) Because everyone has a different trigger for anxiety, it can be difficult to supply a cure that's "one size fits all." Whether your anxiety peaks because of a crowded room or being alone, too much work or not enough, being outside or being indoors, the source of anxiety may seem to be something in the outside world that's agitating something inside you and eliciting a response—but what's *inside* is causing anxious feelings.

Researchers have found that taking 1 tablespoon of coconut oil 1 to 3 times daily can reduce the incidence of anxiety as effectively as some prescription drugs. Some doctors, including New York psychiatrist Kelly Brogan, MD, believe that inflammation in the brain can lead to anxiety and depression. Coconut oil's anti-inflammatory properties, therefore, can reduce brain inflammation while also giving your brain the fuel it needs to function optimally. The oil works by providing medium-chain fatty acids and lauric acid to the brain to aid mental clarity and blood flow. Not only can these elements in coconut oil reduce the physical symptoms of anxiety, they can also help to provide the brain and body with improved functioning that can stop anxiety before it starts.

Anxiety is a response to changes in the brain and environment that result in physical symptoms including heart palpitations, excessive sweating, shortness of breath, nausea, dizziness, and dry mouth. Anxiety works in a cycle that begins with a situation that triggers a mental response that elicits physical symptoms; the symptoms (heart palpitations, sweating, nausea, etc.) worsen the anxiety and exacerbate the physical symptoms. The key to alleviating anxiety is in the brain. By recognizing the trigger, changing the environment, and calming the brain's reaction by identifying the trigger as just that, you can reduce the severity and frequency of anxiety.

THE NEED FOR MEDICAL INTERVENTION

Many people swear by diet for their depression and anxiety needs, and their claims are well supported—treatments using nutrition to combat depression can be very effective. However, a portion of the population that suffers from serious anxiety issues caused by biological dysfunction may need something more. Do not avoid physician intervention when it comes to serious depression issues. If you feel suicidal or notice your anxiety becoming debilitating, seek professional help immediately.

35. TOUGHEN YOUR TEETH

Teeth are made of the same elements as bone, and you need a certain amount of dietary calcium daily in order to keep both your bones and your teeth strong and healthy. Coconut oil helps the body process and utilize calcium, magnesium, and other minerals that are needed for maintaining and strengthening teeth, and ensures proper absorption of these minerals into the blood stream and tissues. The oil's antiviral, antibacterial properties also help to prevent illnesses and disease caused by the viruses, bacteria, and germs that are ever present in the mouth.

TO STRENGTHEN AND MAINTAIN THE HEALTH OF YOUR TEETH, USE:

1 to 3 tablespoons of coconut oil

Ingest every day, by itself or in your food. (See also "'Pull' Bacteria from Your Mouth" in Chapter 4.)

The foods you consume improve or reduce the health of your teeth. If your diet supplies the nutrients your body needs, the structure of your teeth is maintained. If your diet is lacking in the necessary nutrients, your body uses the nutrients available for other body processes, leaving your teeth to suffer. When serious deficiencies occur, the body can actually turn to areas (like the teeth) that have a concentration of needed minerals and degrade those areas of minerals for use elsewhere. For instance, if you are deficient in calcium and magnesium, your body can degrade the quality of your teeth and use those minerals in any of the chemical and systematic processes for survival.

Coconut oil helps assist the body in utilizing the building blocks provided by your diet, while also safeguarding the health of your teeth. As you can see, the value of a quality diet rich in nutrient-dense whole foods is also imperative in maintaining healthy teeth.

36. REPEL INSECTS

Bug bites and stings aren't just an annoyance. A growing number of serious illnesses and diseases can result from the transmission of microbes by bugs, and severe infections can occur at the site of a bite or sting after the skin has been irritated and left open to infections. Although applying a commercial bug repellant may seem like the simple solution, concerns about potentially harmful chemical ingredients such as DEET (currently used in more than 200 bug repellant products) are leading more and more people to seek natural methods of safeguarding their skin from insect bites and stings. Luckily, you can make a simple, safe, effective insect repellant by blending coconut oil—with its immunity-boosting and illness-preventing properties provided by lauric and capric acids—and insect-repelling tea tree oil (a natural derivative of the melaleuca plant).

TO MAKE ½ CUP OF THIS ALL-NATURAL BUG REPELLANT, COMBINE:

½ cup coconut oil, warmed to liquefy
10 drops tea tree oil

Blend ingredients together. Pour into a spray bottle. Apply directly to your skin as often as necessary to prevent bug bites and stings.

Coconut oil's antibacterial and antiviral properties also offer topical protection against bacteria, germs, and viruses that can breed on your skin's surface or cause festering every time you scratch a bug bite. Tea tree oil also offers antiseptic benefits that can fight infection and skin irritation. This potent combination helps safeguard you from the possible discomforts and illnesses that can result from bug bites and stings, while providing intense moisturizing benefits to improve your skin's health at the same time.

37. GET HEALTHY PROTEIN WITH COCONUT BRAISED BEEF

This hearty dish is unlike any beef recipe you've ever tried before. Tender and tantalizing, its unique combination of flavorings will bring to mind the cuisines of the Caribbean, India, South America, and the Pacific Islands.

THIS PROTEIN-PACKED DISH WITH A RICH, CARAMEL-COLORED SAUCE SERVES 6. COCONUT, LIME, GINGER, AND HOT CHILIES GIVE IT A SPICY-SWEET, EXOTIC FLAVOR.

2 hot dried red chilies

3 cloves garlic, minced

1 (1-inch piece) ginger, grated

1 tablespoon chili powder

Juice and zest of 2 limes

2 tablespoons coconut oil

2 pounds stewing beef

1 (13.5-ounce) can coconut milk

Sea salt, to taste

In a food processor, place chilies, garlic, ginger, chili powder, and lime juice and zest; process until finely chopped.

In a heavy-bottomed skillet, heat coconut oil over medium-high heat. Add spice paste from the food processor; cook, stirring occasionally, for about 2 minutes.

Add stewing beef to skillet; cook for about 5 minutes, or until browned.

Pour in coconut milk; bring mixture to a boil. Reduce heat to low and cover; allow mixture to simmer, stirring occasionally, for about 1½ hours, or until meat is extremely tender.

Remove lid and cook for another 10 to 15 minutes, stirring frequently, until sauce is thick and caramel colored.

Add salt, and serve with rice.

38. FIGHT FUNGAL INFECTIONS

For fighting fungal infections, coconut oil's natural healing capabilities exceed those of products provided at your local drugstore—in fact, a study published in the *Journal of Medicinal Food* in June 2007 advised that "Coconut oil should be used in the treatment of fungal infections." When the body succumbs to a fungal infection, a number of possible afflictions may arise, ranging from mild discomfort and fever to severe bouts of infection that spread to other parts of the body (even the brain, lungs, and internal organs), requiring hospitalization—some of these afflictions may even result in death. According to a 2013 article in *ScienceDaily (www.sciencedaily.com/ releases/2013/12/131223181303.htm)*, fungal infections cause more than 1.3 million deaths worldwide annually. You can greatly reduce your chances of having a bout of life-altering or life-threatening illness related to a fungal infection, however, and coconut oil can play a role.

TO HELP PREVENT AGAINST FUNGAL INFECTIONS, USE:

1 to 3 tablespoons of coconut oil

Consume each day (neat or added to food).

TO TOPICALLY AID FUNGAL INFECTIONS, USE:

1 teaspoon of coconut oil

With a cotton ball, apply coconut oil to the affected area of the skin as often as 5 to 10 times per day.

More than half the composition of coconut oil is a saturated fat that belongs to the classification of medium-chain fatty acids. This part of the coconut oil is processed by the liver and broken down to create lauric acid, which in turn becomes an antibacterial, antimicrobial, antiviral, and antifungal combatant against infection. These powerful properties of coconut oil can effectively relieve fungal infections.

39. REGULATE CANDIDA

Many people have had a yeast infection that resulted from candida overgrowth. Candida is not an isolated fungus that only creates the vaginal condition with which so many women are familiar. It can also affect any part of the skin and the digestive, respiratory, or urinary tract, thriving in dark, damp areas that have enough heat to allow bacteria to grow. This means that feet, lungs, and even scalps are susceptible to fungal infections resulting from candida overgrowth.

An overgrowth of candida commonly results from lifestyle factors such as diet (especially one high in sugar and carbohydrates), prescription drugs (specifically antibiotics), alcohol intake, oral contraceptives, and stress. In addition to managing these factors, you can minimize your chances of experiencing a candida overgrowth by adding coconut oil to your daily regimen. Scientific studies performed at Nigeria's University College Hospital and published in the *Journal of Medicinal Food* found that coconut oil's antifungal properties were active in combatting candida, and recommended using the oil "in the treatment of fungal infections in view of emerging drug-resistant *Candida* species."

TO HELP SPEED RECOVERY FROM A CANDIDA OVERGROWTH, USE:

Coconut oil as needed

Apply coconut oil topically to the infected area multiple times per day. You can also ingest 1 to 3 tablespoons of coconut oil per day, either by the spoonful or in your food. Here's a delicious salad dressing that's packed with healthy ingredients to improve digestion and help combat candida.

TO MAKE 20 1½-OUNCE SERVINGS OF THIS GINGER SALAD DRESSING, COMBINE:

2 tablespoon sliced ginger
3 garlic cloves
1 tablespoon honey
¼ cup Bragg Liquid Aminos or soy sauce
½ cup coconut oil
¼ cup sesame oil
⅓ cup rice vinegar
Optional: ¼ cup water

Combine all ingredients except water in a high-speed blender.

Blend until all ingredients are emulsified. Add water as needed while blending to reach desired taste and consistency. Store dressing in an airtight container in the refrigerator for up to a week.

40. TREAT THRUSH

Thrush is an oral condition caused by an overgrowth of the candida fungus when the normal balance of ever-present bacteria in the mouth gets upset. Thrush most commonly affects infants and young children. The symptoms of thrush include the physical appearance of white, slightly raised sores in the mouth that can sometimes resemble cottage cheese. Although the condition can be uncomfortable, with sores that bleed when irritated by eating or brushing teeth, severe cases that affect the esophagus and digestive system are very rare. Hormone fluctuations and medications such as corticosteroids can contribute to an upset in the normal levels of candida, resulting in thrush. Thrush is most commonly treated with antifungal medications, but it can be relieved effectively and naturally with coconut oil due to the oil's fast-acting antifungal properties.

ADULTS SHOULD USE:

1 to 3 tablespoons of coconut oil

Consume daily, by itself or in food.

TO AID CHILDREN:

Coconut oil as needed

Apply topically by putting coconut oil on a cotton swab and coating the child's mouth, gums, inside cheeks, and lips repeatedly every day until the overgrowth is normalized.

Coconut oil contains a composition of saturated fat molecules called medium-chain fatty acids. During the digestion of these medium-chain fatty acids, the body produces lauric acid, which acts as an antibacterial, antiviral, antimicrobial, and antifungal agent. In addition to the coconut oil regimen, infants, children, and adults can benefit from ingesting a probiotic that improves digestion by balancing the "good bacteria" in the intestines to help fight candida overgrowth. Live culture probiotics can be found in yogurt, kefir, and a number of refrigerated products at supermarkets and health-food stores; probiotic supplements are also available at many vitamin retailers as well as online.

41. FIGHT YEAST INFECTIONS

The sudden and excruciatingly itchy, burning pain associated with yeast infections is a very unique sensation that makes many women rush for over-the-counter and prescription treatments that promise to destroy the infection and deliver pain relief. Instead of using powerful, chemical-laden pills or messy creams, however, you have the perfect natural remedy in your kitchen cabinet: coconut oil. Coconut oil has antifungal and probiotic properties that can help to rid your body of the yeast infection caused by candida overgrowth (see "Regulate Candida" earlier in this chapter). The anti-inflammatory and antihistamine benefits in the oil's lauric acid can also relieve pain and itching by minimizing the spread of the infection and relieving the inflammation internally.

TO HELP REMEDY THE YEAST INFECTION INTERNALLY, USE:

3 to 5 tablespoons of coconut oil

Ingest every day. Also see the following section "Apply Topical Relief for Yeast Infections" for ways to use topical applications.

Dairy products can exacerbate yeast problems, so you may opt to eliminate them from your diet, at least temporarily until the condition improves. Here's a delightful recipe for a dairy-free "cream" topping that complements both sweet and savory dishes.

TO MAKE 2 CUPS OF THIS RICH COCONUT CREAM TOPPING, COMBINE:

2 cups coconut oil
1 tablespoon powdered sugar or 1 tablespoon of your favorite seasoning
Salt to taste

In a large mixing bowl, beat coconut oil on high until stiff peaks form. Gradually add sugar or spices and salt while beating until stiff peaks form. Serve atop your favorite dish.

42. APPLY TOPICAL RELIEF FOR YEAST INFECTIONS

As we discussed in previous entries, coconut oil offers a reliable way to help prevent and treat yeast infections. Every tablespoon you consume will aid in attacking the infection at its source (in your gut and urinary tract) in four ways:

1. Its antifungal property fights the infection.
2. Its probiotic property promotes the growth of good bacteria needed to regulate candida. Coconut oil's lauric acid and capric acid help to deliver relief from yeast infections by boosting your body's ability to fight the infection and warding off future infections.
3. They provide anti-inflammatory and antihistamine properties that reduce the itching and burning sensation.
4. They slightly numb the area to ease discomfort.

Don't limit the benefits you can gain from coconut oil by merely drinking it. To help your yeast infection subside, use the oil topically as well. You can ease the itching and burning sensations that result from a yeast infection internally by soaking a tampon (removed from its applicator) in liquid coconut oil until saturated and inserting it into your vagina for two to four hours. Then remove the tampon, discard it, and repeat the process as needed. (If symptoms continue longer than thirty-six to forty-eight hours, seek medical attention.) This one-two punch delivers the necessary assistance your body needs to reduce the candida overgrowth and return your system to normal.

43. SPEED UTI RECOVERY

A urinary tract infection (commonly referred to as a UTI) is a bacterial infection that occurs in the areas that make up the urinary tract: the bladder, kidneys, and the tube that connects them. A UTI starts as an infection of the bladder. Bacteria adhere to the walls of the urinary tract and usually produce symptoms such as pain when urinating, foul-smelling and cloudy urine, and possibly pain in the abdomen and kidneys. Caused by germs infecting the area of your urinary tract, a UTI can be brought on by holding urine too long, wiping from back to front after urinating, or not urinating immediately after sex.

TRY THE FOLLOWING DRINK TO EASE DISCOMFORT AND SPEED RECOVERY FROM A UTI:

½ cup unsweetened cranberry juice (pure cranberry juice, not cranberry cocktail)
1 tablespoon coconut oil
4 ounces water

Combine ingredients and stir to mix well; drink as often as you choose. Cranberry juice contains substances that keep the UTI-causing germs from sticking to the walls of the urinary tract. With the pain-relieving and bacteria-fighting properties of coconut oil, this drink helps shorten healing time and minimize symptoms associated with a UTI.

A bladder infection can be remedied by antibacterial medications, and there are a number of over-the-counter UTI treatments—but you can effectively rid yourself of the infection and minimize the resulting symptoms naturally by ingesting coconut oil. Coconut oil's antimicrobial and antibacterial properties kill the germs and bacteria that cause a UTI, making the oil an effective preventative. If the bladder infection is accompanied by fever, chills, nausea, and vomiting, the infection has progressed to a kidney infection, which is far more dangerous and should be treated immediately by a professional.

44. PREVENT NOSEBLEEDS

Nosebleeds, though not a hazard to your health, can be messy, embarrassing, and annoying. They may be caused by a number of conditions, ranging from trauma to high blood pressure to inherited membrane thinness, but allergy reactions and/or inflammation due to allergies are the most common causes of chronic nosebleeds. Nosebleeds often result from excessive dryness in the nasal cavity, which causes the blood vessels in the nose to become easily agitated and burst, resulting in the outpouring of blood from the nasal cavities.

To help prevent nosebleeds, try a not-so-new method that is growing in popularity because of its natural healing properties and effectiveness: coconut oil. With its many health-promoting elements, including lauric and capric acids that reduce inflammation and irritation while also boosting immunity, coconut oil helps to eliminate the causes of nosebleeds. Use coconut oil topically as well as ingesting it daily as a preventative.

TO PROVIDE RELIEF TOPICALLY, USE:

Coconut oil as needed

Moisten a cotton swab with coconut oil and swab the inside of the nose in order to moisturize tissues and relieve dryness that can contribute to nosebleeds. The oil's antihistamine properties reduce inflammation of the nasal cavities and provide allergy-symptom relief.

TO STRENGTHEN THE HEALTH OF THE MEMBRANES IN THE NOSE, USE:

1 to 3 tablespoons of coconut oil for adults or ½ to 1 tablespoon for children per day

Consume daily, alone or in food, to promote a quality blood supply to the area.

Coconut oil is natural and gentle enough to be consumed even by infants and children. It also improves immunity and prevents sinus and nasal infections, which can reduce the incidence of nosebleeds.

DON'T TIP THE HEAD BACK!

When dealing with a nosebleed, a common reaction is to tilt the head back and plug the nose. This is *not* a recommended treatment method, though, because it keeps the blood inside the nose and forces it back into the sinuses.

45. ELIMINATE LICE

If you have schoolchildren you're probably familiar with lice—they can infest the scalps of multiple children in a matter of a few days. Because the itchy symptoms can take weeks or even months to develop, it can be difficult to pinpoint when, where, and how the initial contraction of lice occurred. Regardless of the source, the most important thing is to resolve the issue as quickly as possible by following this treatment sequence:

1. Kill the lice.
2. Rid the head of the eggs.
3. Thoroughly wash the clothes, bedding, and sleeping area of the infested person(s) to reduce the chance of a future infestation and to protect everyone in the household.

Instead of using over-the-counter lice treatments that include powerful chemicals, opt for a natural method to kill lice instead.

1. Rinse the scalp with apple cider vinegar, allowing vinegar to dry on the hair.
2. Comb out eggs and nits as much as possible.
3. Combine 1 cup of coconut oil and 2 tablespoons each of anise essential oil and ylang-ylang essential oil
4. Coat the hair completely, cover with plastic wrap, and allow the solution to set for 12 to 18 hours to suffocate the nits.
5. Rinse hair and wash thoroughly with shampoo.
6. Comb the hair thoroughly using a lice comb in order to remove the nits and eggs as effectively as possible. If necessary, repeat the process again until no lice remain.

Anise and ylang-ylang essential oils contain antibacterial, antifungal, and insecticidal properties. In a study published in October 2002 in the *Israel Medical Association Journal*, 119 schoolchildren infected with head lice were treated with a combination of coconut oil and these two essential oils—with a 92 percent success rate.

PREVENT LICE INFILTRATION

Because school-aged children are exposed to a number of other kids every day in the classroom setting, it is absolutely essential that you safeguard their heads (and your home) with lice-prevention methods:

- Use apple cider vinegar rinses.
- Keep hair pulled back.
- Use hairspray to prevent lice.
- Regularly check your child's head for lice, nits, or eggs.

46. IMPROVE SLEEP QUALITY

Our minds and bodies are profoundly affected by the amount and quality of our sleep. Two surveys conducted by the American Cancer Society found that people who slept seven hours per night had a greater likelihood of living longer than those who slept more or less. If you have trouble falling asleep or staying asleep, coconut oil can help you achieve the quality rest you've always dreamed of. The oil's aromatherapy benefits, plus the anti-inflammatory benefits provided by the lauric acid when used topically on the skin, aid the process of mentally preparing you to go to sleep.

AS A TOPICAL SLEEP AID, USE:

Coconut oil as needed
Optional: a few drops of lavender essential oil

Dab coconut oil, alone or in combination with other calming essential oils such as lavender, chamomile, or vanilla, to the insides of your wrists and at your temples to help you sleep more soundly.

Ingesting coconut oil also helps to regulate the body's blood flow and metabolism, improve digestion, and minimize anxiety—all of which can enhance your quality of sleep. By consuming 1 to 3 tablespoons of coconut oil per day, you can maximize the benefits provided by the plentiful phytochemicals and the unique combination of lauric and capric acids, and wake well rested every morning.

"WINDING DOWN" IS ESSENTIAL TO GOOD SLEEP

If you lie down to sleep, only to have your head flooded with thoughts, ideas, or worries, you may find it beneficial to start a "winding down" regimen before bedtime. During the hour before you plan to sleep, avoid cleaning, writing e-mails, or watching or reading anything over-stimulating. Surround yourself with low lighting, soothing music, and other relaxing elements that will allow you to fall asleep and stay asleep.

47. EAT VEGGIE SOUP WITH COCONUT OIL TO EASE COLDS

The tantalizing aromas of garlic and onion, the spicy kick of cayenne, and the vibrant colors of red lentils and deep green spinach make this Spicy Red Lentil Spinach Soup a treat for the senses. Let it take the chill off a winter night or help to relieve a common cold. Coconut oil's antibacterial properties can ease cold symptoms, while spinach's many vitamins—including A, C, E, K, B_2, and B_6—nourish body and mind.

TO MAKE 8 SERVINGS OF THIS FLAVORFUL, VEGAN SOUP COMBINE:

1 cup coconut oil

1 cup onion, diced

2 cloves garlic, minced

1 teaspoon garlic powder

½ teaspoon cayenne pepper

4 cups vegetable stock

2 cups red lentils

2 cups spinach leaves

Salt to taste

In a large pot over medium heat, heat coconut oil for 5 minutes.

Add onions and minced garlic to the pot and stir to sweat, about 5 to 7 minutes.

Sprinkle onions and garlic with garlic powder and cayenne, and stir for 1 minute.

Add vegetable stock and lentils to the pot. Cover, reduce heat to simmer, and simmer for 30 minutes.

Add spinach to the pot and stir until leaves are wilted. Season with salt to taste.

48. MAKE A NATURAL MASSAGE OIL

A massage should be a calming, enjoyable experience that allows you to relax and recharge. The type of massage oil you choose to use can either soothe or stimulate you, depending on its ingredients. Basically, a massage oil should provide the lubrication necessary to prevent friction during the rubbing and kneading process, plus added skin-moisturizing benefits. Coconut oil does both—and more.

TRY THIS SIMPLE, AROMATIC RECIPE— YOU'LL NEVER USE A COMMERCIAL MASSAGE OIL AGAIN!

1 cup coconut oil, warmed to liquefy
Several drops of your preferred essential oil, or a combination of oils

Pour 1 cup of coconut oil into a bowl. Add essential oil(s) to the coconut oil and stir well to blend. Massage oil blend into the skin—or better yet, have a professional massage therapist or a loved one give you a luscious, healthy massage using your special concoction.

The refreshing, tropical scent of coconut oil by itself instantly puts you in a pleasant mood—but consider adding fragrant, essential oils that trigger relaxation or uplift your mood, such as lavender, bergamot, lemongrass, sweet orange, vanilla, or ylang-ylang. Coconut oil is the perfect "carrier oil" (meaning it blends well with essential oils that are too strong to apply to the skin without diluting them). Its lauric and capric acids combine to provide powerful and effective antibacterial, antiviral, and antimicrobial properties that also protect the skin from possible illnesses and diseases.

Many commonly used massage oils contain chemicals and additives that can elicit skin reactions and irritations, or even promote the growth of bacteria and germs on the skin. However, you can make your own gentle, all-natural, inexpensive massage oil that's a delight to use and nourishing to your skin—without risk of unwanted side effects.

49. SPEED PERINEUM HEALING

The perineum is the sensitive area of skin between the vagina and anus. In the weeks building up to labor and the birth of a baby, midwives or OBs often recommend massaging the area frequently in preparation for the stretching that occurs during delivery. This helps reduce or prevent the tearing that commonly occurs as the baby exits the birth canal. Not only is this tearing uncomfortable in such a sensitive area, it can lead to festering or infection because the perineum is easily exposed to bacteria. Coconut oil is a wonderfully soothing skin-softener, so it's the perfect product for this personal massage. Plus coconut oil's multiple antibacterial benefits naturally fight germs and help prevent infection. Apply coconut oil to the perineum regularly, not only before delivery for preparation purposes, but also following the birth to speed healing and stave off infection.

In the days leading up to delivery and after the baby's birth, use 1 teaspoon to 1 tablespoon of coconut oil to massage the perineum gently as often as needed. The oil's lauric acid has antibacterial, antiviral, and antimicrobial properties that protect against illness and infection in new moms. Its anti-inflammatory properties that reduce swelling and pain at the sight of the perineum also comfort the trauma caused by birth.

TO REDUCE INFLAMMATION IN THE DAYS AFTER THE BIRTH OF A BABY, USE:

1 teaspoon to 1 tablespoon of coconut oil

Apply to the site regularly throughout the day, as needed, to reduce inflammation, prevent infection, and speed healing time, naturally.

50. INCREASE MOTHER'S MILK SUPPLY

Not surprisingly, diet is one of the most important factors in the health of a new mom and her baby. If you plan to nurse your baby, consuming a diet rich in healthy fats and whole foods that provide an abundance of protein and complex carbohydrates will help you to produce an abundance of quality breastmilk. Coconut oil's distinctive, medium-chain fatty acids provide an ample supply of the dietary fat your body needs in the production of breastmilk—in fact, coconut oil's lauric acid is also found in breastmilk.

Rich in lutein and lauric acid, coconut oil also offers antibacterial, antiviral, and antimicrobial benefits to safeguard the health of mom and baby by improving immunity and fighting possible infections. Few other products can honestly make these claims, while also providing healthy fat to the new mother's diet, thus improving the quality and quantity of breastmilk for even the hungriest of babies. New moms can consume 1 to 3 tablespoons of coconut oil daily, either by itself or in food.

Of course, other factors such as stress and sleep quality can negatively affect the amount of breastmilk produced, so it is imperative that you focus on a lifestyle that provides stress relief, adequate sleep, minimal energy expenditure, and a diet rich in nutrient-dense foods.

INCREASING MOM'S MILK SUPPLY WITH ALCOHOL?

A well-known old wives' tale for increasing the milk supply recommends that new moms drink alcohol to hasten the milk-ejection reflex (sometimes called "let-down"). Recent research shows that it is not the alcohol but the calming effect produced by the alcohol on the mother's parasympathetic nervous system that allows the milk to release. Following delivery, use proven relaxation techniques rather than alcohol to safeguard your baby from possible alcohol contamination in your breastmilk.

51. ELIMINATE EAR INFECTIONS

Flaring red with irritation, infected ears are uncomfortable and difficult to treat. Recurring ear infections are often treated with antibiotics—they may even require surgery, especially in very young children, in order to relieve the pressure of multiple ear infections and refrain from excessive antibiotic treatments. The lauric acid produced by the medium-chain fatty acids found in coconut oil is a little-known, yet extremely effective, aid for ear infections.

Acting as a powerful combatant against microbes, bacteria, viruses, and fungi, the lauric acid produced by coconut oil is the perfect natural remedy for earaches. Coconut oil can be either ingested or used topically to treat and prevent ear infections— or both. To promote immunity and combat infections internally:

- Adults should consume 1 to 3 tablespoons of coconut oil per day.
- Children should consume between ½ to 1 tablespoon of coconut oil per day.

Coconut oil can be consumed in its liquid or solid state. Ingest it by itself or mix it in with other food or drinks as part of a recipe.

AS A TOPICAL TREATMENT FOR EAR INFECTIONS, USE:

½ tablespoon of slightly liquefied coconut oil

Drip into the ear and let the oil remain in place for 5 to 10 minutes. This treatment can be applied 2 to 6 times per day.

52. REMOVE EARWAX SAFELY

Any physician will tell you that your ears naturally cleanse themselves and require no additional treatment to keep them free of excess wax buildup. If you speak to audiologists about maintaining your ear health, they will undoubtedly warn you against using cotton swabs or any other type of instrument to remove possible buildup because, when inserting anything small into the ear's canal, you might damage the internal ear. So what can you do to get rid of excess wax without using over-the-counter products that contain potentially harmful chemicals?

Coconut oil provides a safe, all-natural, and effective option that not only delivers results, but does so without unwanted side effects. Additionally, coconut oil's health-boosting properties act to kill bacteria, fungi, viruses, and microbes that can easily turn into ear infections. Try this quick-and-easy process to clean your ears:

1. Warm the oil to a liquid consistency.
2. Pour ½ to 1 tablespoon of coconut oil into your ear, and allow oil to stay there for 10 minutes.
3. Rinse with warm water. This allows the excess earwax to break down and flow out, without any damage to the ear. Coconut oil, with lauric acid's germ-fighting power, also provides protection from infection or irritation.

Some people produce more earwax than others, and many have tried over-the-counter remedies that include flushes, aquatic pulsation, or manual excavating processes. These treatments can alleviate buildup initially but quickly create a problem when the body, in reaction to the earwax removal, produces even more wax, causing more buildup. Coconut oil eliminates the need for any instruments, synthetic treatments, or expensive medical procedures to cleanse your ears.

53. RELIEVE STRESS WITH AROMATHERAPY

Not only can coconut oil provide physical health benefits when you add it to your diet, this powerful oil can also have a major impact on your mental and emotional states. Earlier in this chapter, we discussed its ability to sharpen mental clarity, relieve depression, and alleviate anxiety. Coconut oil's powerful phytochemicals and its potent lauric and capric acids also help to combat stress, improve focus, and stabilize your moods. In addition to ingesting it daily, you can inhale its aroma to soothe your body, mind, and emotions.

If you know something about aromatherapy, you know that scents trigger all sorts of reactions in the brain. We associate the aroma of coconut oil with the salubrious, sun-drenched environment of the tropics, as well as with serenity, pleasure, and relaxation. Applying coconut oil to your skin not only lets you enjoy its aromatherapy benefits, it also provides effective and intensive moisturizing therapy. Your body's natural heat will intensify the aroma of the coconut oil. However, only virgin coconut oil contains aromatherapy properties—fractionated oils used in many commercial products have been stripped of some of their innate qualities, including scent.

Apply ample amounts of coconut oil (neat or blended with essential oils) to your skin multiple times per day. Give special attention to the sensitive points behind your ear lobes, at your temples, and on the insides of your wrists where blood flow is most prominent. Your body's heat and circulation will make the aroma more pronounced. You may also want to add specific essential oils that can ease stress, such as lavender, lemongrass, chamomile, or clary sage. Coconut oil is the ideal carrier oil with which to blend potent and expensive essential oils for safe, practical, topical application.

54. ALLEVIATE ARTHRITIS DISCOMFORT

When was the last time you heard an arthritis sufferer exclaim that he was cured with an all-natural remedy . . . or even cured at all? According to the Centers for Disease Control, nearly 23 percent of adults in the United States and half of those over the age of sixty-five have been diagnosed with arthritis. If you're one of the millions who suffer from the pain and limited mobility of arthritis, you don't have to rely on prescription drugs that may be minimally effective or might even cause major side effects. Coconut oil's powerful, naturally occurring anti-inflammatory properties, when added to your daily regimen, can have remarkable positive effects on the health of your joints. Try this double-whammy to help relieve suffering:

1. Consume 1 to 3 tablespoon of all-natural coconut oil every day, either by itself or in food.
2. Apply coconut oil directly to uncomfortable joints to maximize benefits and speed healing.

In a number of studies performed to test the effectiveness of coconut oil on inflammatory conditions such as arthritis and rheumatoid arthritis, researchers found that polyphenolics isolated from virgin coconut oil inhibited adjuvant-induced arthritis in rats through antioxidant and anti-inflammatory action. One study, published in the journal *International Immunopharmacology* in 2014, found that the antioxidants in the oil actually reduced inflammation in arthritic rats more effectively than an often-prescribed anti-inflammatory drug.

With immunity-building properties from lauric acid and capric acid that help to maintain your overall quality of health, coconut oil can also provide protection against unwanted illnesses and conditions that can aggravate arthritis. Whether you apply coconut oil topically or ingest it, you needn't fear possible side effects that can result from the pharmaceutical treatments often recommended for arthritis.

55. BOOST HEALTH WITH BEETS AND COCONUT OIL

Beets are one of the healthiest foods you can eat. The nitrates in beets, which convert to nitric oxide in your body, may be the reason this veggie can help lower blood pressure. The betaine fights inflammation and protects your cells. The phytonutrients that make beets red may also help fight cancer. Plus beets provide vitamin C to boost your immune system, potassium to aid nerves and muscles, manganese for healthy bones, and lots more. This colorful recipe combines beets' amazing health benefits with the antibacterial, anti-inflammatory, and antifungal properties of coconut oil. Whipped up with cashews and chickpeas for protein and texture, it offers a tempting, slightly sweet spin on traditional hummus.

AS A SPREAD ON PITAS OR A DIP FOR CHIPS, THIS BEAUTIFUL BEET HUMMUS MAKES 16 SERVINGS.

2 cups chickpeas, drained

2 red beets, peeled and greens removed

⅛ cup lemon juice

½ cup cashews

2 cloves garlic, peeled

¼ cup coconut oil

Salt to taste

Combine all ingredients except coconut oil in a blender.

Blend on high, adding coconut oil while blending until desired consistency is achieved.

Move hummus from blender to a serving dish and sprinkle with salt to taste.

Although beets don't rank at the top of everyone's list of favorite foods, this pretty and healthful dish will surely change the way some people feel about beets.

PART 2

BEAUTY AND PERSONAL CARE

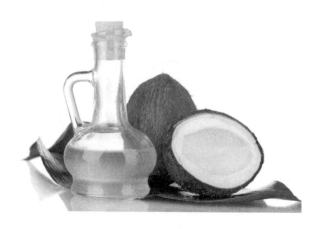

Chapter 3

SKIN CARE

The skin is your body's largest organ. It's also your body's first line of defense again environmental toxins, germs, and other hazards. It provides a physical barrier that prevents microorganisms from getting inside your body, where they can cause infection or other problems. Every day, your skin is exposed to pathogens, wind, cold, damaging UV rays from the sun, and much more—and it does a remarkable job of protecting you. This monumental task, however, takes a toll on your skin.

You can help to safeguard your skin from both natural and manmade risks—even those that may lurk in substances designed for use on your skin, including some beauty and personal care products. Your skin-protection regimen should be one that both proactively protects your skin from pathogens and environmental damage, and also nurtures your skin's health. One easy, inexpensive, all-natural way to do this is with coconut oil. In this section of *Coconut Oil for Health* you'll learn ways to safely apply coconut oil to your skin to treat conditions such as psoriasis and acne, soothe sunburn, prevent skin infections, minimize stretch marks, and lots more. This amazing oil can also prevent irritation and redness from abrasive or chemical treatments due to the anti-inflammatory benefits of its lauric and capric acids. It also provides collagen-building, restorative nutrients that deliver anti-aging benefits you can see and feel! Want to reduce the incidence of fine lines and wrinkles, age spots and areas of discoloration, or even athlete's foot and rough patches of skin? Coconut oil offers help for all these complaints.

When you use coconut oil for your skin-care regimen, you need not fear unpleasant side effects and unwanted results. Just follow the easy instructions outlined in this chapter. Regardless of your age or skin type, coconut oil can give you the results you desire with the safety you need.

56. PROTECT YOUR SKIN AGAINST EVERYDAY BACTERIA

Germs lurk everywhere—on door handles, the keypad at your local supermarket, the swing set at your children's school playground. Fear of infection is causing millions of people to avoid the long-standing tradition of greeting someone with a handshake. The most common product used today to combat bacterial infections or illnesses that may be picked up by such everyday contacts is the antibacterial hand-sanitizer. However, many of these over-the-counter products use powerful chemicals or alcohol to eliminate bacteria on the skin—which can also kill off the beneficial bacteria that safeguard your health against common illnesses.

If you're looking for an effective, all-natural alternative to the commercial antibacterial sanitizers, look no further than coconut oil—it has been used for centuries to protect against illnesses and diseases. Packed with naturally occurring lauric and capric acids that can bolster your immunity against infection, coconut oil helps restore a natural balance of beneficial bacteria that can strengthen your immunity, while also killing harmful bacteria.

1. Rub ½ tablespoon coconut oil directly on your skin—especially your hands and face, which are always exposed and where bacteria can thrive—as often as desired to help protect against infection and illness.
2. Allow the oil to be absorbed into the skin for 5 to 10 minutes.

Coconut oil effectively kills "bad" bacteria, provides your skin with a barrier of protection, and moisturizes your skin—in one simple step.

57. SOOTHE DRY SKIN

So many conditions can contribute to dry skin that it's difficult to find someone who *doesn't* suffer from this condition. Do you wash your hands repeatedly throughout the day to prevent potential infection? Are you exposed to extremely cool or dry conditions because of your climate? Do you suffer from a skin condition that is exacerbated by lifestyle or environmental factors? Do hormonal issues upset your skin's pH balance? Coconut oil can help relieve dry skin and repair the effects of dryness while also delivering the germ-fighting properties of lauric acid and capric acid that safeguard your skin's health.

Uncomfortable dry skin can affect any part of your body. Not only do you want to get rid of dry patches on your skin, you want a dry-skin soother that also provides protection from infections caused by bacteria, viruses, fungi, and microbes that can attack the vulnerable areas of the skin that have become cracked and irritated by dryness. Coconut oil delivers intensive moisturizing benefits, while simultaneously providing antibacterial, antiviral support for damaged skin.

1. Apply a thin layer of coconut oil to dry patches of skin.
2. Allow the oil to be absorbed into the skin for 5 to 10 minutes.
3. Reapply the oil as often as needed.

Your skin is the largest organ in your body, and you can give it support by consuming just 1 to 3 tablespoons of coconut oil daily. This helps your body to better absorb and deliver essential nutrients needed for optimal skin health. By maintaining a daily dietary regimen that includes the consumption of coconut oil, you can quickly, easily, and safely improve internal conditions that prevent dry skin and keep your skin moisturized regardless of the external conditions it has to endure.

58. USE AS THE BEST BABY LOTION EVER

When choosing a baby lotion, obviously you don't want one with chemicals, dyes, or perfumes that could possibly irritate your baby's sensitive skin. The sebaceous glands on a baby's skin are designed to keep it supple and moisturized for many months following birth, so usually a baby's skin does not need additional moisturizers or ointments. If skin conditions such as dryness, redness, or irritation do arise, you want the safest option, one that is completely natural, gentle, and minimally processed. You want coconut oil.

Packed with properties that not only reduce inflammation and irritation of the skin, but also provide protective elements that prevent infections and guard against bacteria, viruses, and fungi that commonly create babies' illnesses, coconut oil is one of the most beneficial skin treatments you can use on your baby's skin.

Apply coconut oil to areas of redness or irritation to soothe skin and promote healing. For eczema, rashes, and even the most uncomfortable or persistent diaper rash, rub on coconut oil as often as possible to help alleviate any discomfort and resolve the underlying cause of irritation—regardless of whether the issue is related to excessive dryness or moisture, chronic skin ailments that result from rubbing (especially on the knees of new crawlers), or exposure to harsh conditions such as cold or heat. You can also use the oil as a shampoo and body wash, too. Massage the oil into the skin and scalp, allow the oil to absorb for just a couple of minutes, and then rinse. This gentle cleanser helps deliver essential soothing nutrients, such as vitamin E, that baby's skin can absorb immediately and safely—that's something no chemical-laden commercial product can promise!

59. PREVENT STRETCH MARKS

Whether you're planning to lose weight or are preparing for the growth that comes with pregnancy, you can benefit from a skin-care regimen that includes coconut oil. When the skin has been stretched and then returns to normal size—as it generally does during weight-loss or after the birth of a baby—stretch marks often result. These streaks of hyperpigmentation can be more prominent as a result of heredity, but you can minimize them by routinely applying plenty of moisturizer to areas where stretch marks commonly appear. In order to prevent the occurrence of stretch marks, it is imperative to keep the skin moisturized and well nourished.

Although many commercially available creams and ointments promise to remove stretch marks or reduce their appearance, coconut oil affords a safe, natural, and effective alternative. In addition to its moisturizing benefits, coconut oil adds essential nutrients, including vitamin E, to the skin. And, you can use coconut oil as often as desired without concern for skin irritation or side effects that can result from the overuse of some products. By continually using coconut oil as your everyday moisturizer on areas prone to stretch marks on the stomach, sides of the torso, legs, buttocks, and/or upper arms, you help your skin stay moisturized and retain elasticity throughout the process of stretching during growth or returning to its normal state.

60. MINIMIZE AGE SPOTS

Age spots are unsightly areas of the skin that appear dark and discolored, sometimes called "liver spots" because hyperpigmentation was once believed to indicate inadequate liver functioning. Resulting from hyperpigmentation that occurs with age, possible nutrient deficiencies, and extensive sun exposure, age spots are a common condition experienced by people over the age of thirty.

TO HELP PREVENT AND MINIMIZE THE APPEARANCE OF AGE SPOTS, USE:

Coconut oil as needed

Apply coconut oil directly to the areas of the skin affected by age spots, as often as necessary. In addition, by ingesting 1 to 3 tablespoons of coconut oil daily you can reduce the degree of discoloration—without fear of adversely affecting the surrounding skin.

Coconut oil's naturally occurring lauric and capric acids help the body to internally regulate nutrient absorption and to utilize those nutrients effectively. Because coconut oil is not digested in the liver, it helps to improve the quality and functioning of the body's components and systems without taxing the liver. Therefore, consuming coconut oil can improve liver functioning and the body's processes, naturally.

Many commercial creams and ointments promise to conceal or cure age spots, but if the active ingredients are synthetic chemicals and additives that reduce the appearance of age spots by bleaching the entire area of the skin—not just the darkened spots—you might end up with a whitened area of skin that looks just as obvious and undesirable as the original condition. You may simply replace one unsightly condition for another.

61. TURN BACK THE CLOCK

The search for the Fountain of Youth may lead to coconut oil. The oil's natural ability to enhance collagen production can make you look younger and healthier, without the use of chemicals or medical procedures. One reason is that coconut oil is packed with skin-regenerating nutrients including lauric acid and capric acid that nourish the face, neck, chest, and other parts of the body that most commonly show aging. It can also be safely applied directly to fine lines, wrinkles, and liver spots on the skin, minimizing their appearance in just a matter of days or weeks.

TO HELP YOUR BODY PRODUCE A HEALTHIER BALANCE OF OILS ON THE SKIN'S SURFACE, USE:

1 to 3 tablespoons of coconut oil

Consume each day, alone or in food.

TO USE TOPICALLY:

Coconut oil as needed

Apply coconut oil to your skin 1 to 3 times daily to regenerate collagen, minimize the appearance and development of fine lines and wrinkles, and maintain your skin's elasticity.

When the lipid content of the skin decreases, the skin's surface layer becomes impaired, causing wrinkles, flaking, and dryness to occur, according to *Dermatologic Therapy* and *Skin Research and Technology* journals. Coconut oil's ingredients mimic the skin's lipid content to help support the intercellular-skin matrix. In addition, coconut oil's antibacterial properties help keep your body free of illnesses and diseases that can result in signs of aging.

By combining simple lifestyle changes with the implementation of coconut oil in your daily routine, you can turn back the clock and start seeing results right away! Try the following recommendations to maintain healthy, youthful skin:

- Drink at least 64 ounces of water daily.
- Consume a diet rich in antioxidant-packed whole foods, such as fresh fruits and vegetables.
- Minimize alcohol consumption.
- Quit smoking.
- Protect your skin from sun exposure.
- Keep your face free of dirt and germs.

62. SOOTHE SUNBURN

Sunburn can ruin a day at beach or on the ski slopes, leaving your skin painfully inflamed and extremely sensitive to touch. Overexposure to the sun's rays not only causes a burning irritation that can take days to subside, it also produces possibly harmful changes in the skin that can develop into cancers of the skin. Coconut oil, with its moisturizing and anti-inflammatory properties that can help soothe sunburn, has not only become one of the most effective all-natural ways to turn down the heat, it may also help to prevent skin cancer.

Providing an abundance of nutrients that are absorbed into the skin, coconut oil can be the perfect sunburn soother—and it brings instant results. By utilizing lauric and capric acids, coconut oil can also help calm sunburn pain by reducing the inflammation of the skin that results from overexposure to the sun's UV rays, giving continuous relief for hours. Coconut oil's all-natural properties produce no undesirable side effects, and its capric acid can provide skin-regenerating benefits that actually speed healing.

AS A PREVENTATIVE, USE:

1 to 3 tablespoons of coconut oil

Ingest daily, alone or in food. This internal protection helps safeguard your skin from the potential danger that results from overexposure to the sun.

AS A TOPICAL AID, USE:

Coconut oil as needed

Apply the oil to burned skin as often as needed for relief.

THE DANGERS OF SUN EXPOSURE

With sun exposure comes the risk of cancerous changes at the cellular level. Skin cancer can metastasize quickly into other forms of cancer that affect other areas of the body. Therefore, it is essential to impede the growth of skin cancer and reduce the chance of it spreading. Minimize sun exposure and use sunblock whenever you're exposed to sunlight for longer than ten minutes.

63. NIX ACNE

Acne is a reaction to bacteria that has been absorbed into the skin's cells or that is causing an encapsulated blockage of one of the skin's sebaceous glands or pores. The clogging of the pores, which are responsible for purging bacteria, dirt, grime, and germs that cause irritation, can lead to redness, irritation, black-heads, whiteheads, or acne. Products that contain salicylic acid, a powerful synthetic acid intended to kill bacteria that cause acne, can actually cause more irritation and can lead to other conditions including dryness, overproduction of oils (in response to the dryness), inflammation, and possibly contribute to wrinkles. By opting for a more natural treatment method—coconut oil—you can achieve results that will leave your face acne-free and moisturized, without unpleasant side effects.

With antibacterial properties from lauric acid, coconut oil can be applied directly to the skin of the face and/or body—wherever acne is prevalent. Soak a cotton ball in liquefied coconut oil and apply a light coating of oil to your skin as often as desired. Coconut oil can also assist in maintaining a healthy balance of oils on the skin and keep your skin free of acne-causing bacteria to further minimize the development of acne. An acne study published in the *Journal of Dermatological Science* in 2013 found that lauric acid inhibited bacterial growth and reduced inflammation. This anti-inflammatory property can reduce redness and irritation on the skin where blotches and discoloration occur. Try blending in tea tree, oregano, or rosemary essential oils for added benefits. In just a matter of days you'll start developing evenly toned, radiant, acne-free skin.

64. REDUCE BODY ACNE

Acne doesn't show up only on the face. Environmental factors and an unhealthy diet wreak havoc with your skin and can cause it to react by producing unsightly body acne: redness, irritation, and/or raised pimples, most commonly appearing on the chest, back, or arms. Acne doesn't just affect teens, either. According to Miami dermatologist Jonette Keri, MD, PhD, nearly 30 percent of adult women and 20 percent of men suffer from breakouts.

By adding coconut oil to your daily skin-care routine, you can maximize your skin's health and reduce the chance of irritation and the development of body acne. When your body breaks down coconut oil, it creates lauric acid, which can combat the bacteria that produce acne.

TO BOOST YOUR BODY'S IMMUNITY, USE:

1 to 3 tablespoons of coconut oil

Ingest daily to improve the natural balance of good and bad bacteria that are released through your skin. This also helps to regulate your body's oil production.

TO PROVIDE TOPICAL BENEFITS, USE:

Coconut oil as needed

Spot-treat areas of body acne using a cotton ball saturated with liquefied coconut oil. This helps minimize the development of bacteria on your skin's surface, eliminate the acne-causing germs and environmental toxins that settle on the skin, and improve the natural balance of oils on the skin's surface.

Additionally, you can improve the quality of your skin by:

- Eating a quality diet rich in nutrient-dense foods, low in sugar, and with an optimal balance of healthy fats and oils.
- Washing your skin regularly to protect against dirt, grime, and naturally occurring oils that can build up in the skin's pores.

65. FEED YOUR SKIN WITH COCONUT BEER-BATTER SHRIMP

You've heard the expression "you are what you eat." When it comes to your skin, this is certainly the case. This recipe is a delicious way to add coconut oil to your diet. The combination of coconut oil and coconut flakes gives the shrimp a distinctive flavor and texture.

THIS RECIPE MAKES ENOUGH COCONUT BEER-BATTER SHRIMP TO SERVE 6 AS A HEALTHY SNACK, OR 4 FOR A MEAL.

3 cups coconut oil for frying

1 egg

¾ cup all-purpose flour, separated

⅔ cup beer

1½ teaspoons baking powder

2 cups coconut flakes

24 shrimp, tails intact

Heat a skillet with 3 cups of coconut oil.

In a bowl, combine egg, ½ cup of flour, beer, and baking powder.

Pour remaining ¼ cup of flour into a second bowl, and coconut flakes into a third.

Holding shrimp by their tails, individually dredge them in flour, dip them into batter, and roll in coconut flakes.

Place shrimp in oil and cook for 2 to 3 minutes before turning and cooking for an additional 2 to 3 minutes, or until they're golden brown.

Remove shrimp and place on a paper towel to collect excess oil. Cool for 2 to 3 minutes, and serve.

66. SOOTHE PSORIASIS AND ECZEMA

Psoriasis and eczema are two immune system skin conditions that can appear as itchy, red, scaly blotches caused by inflammation. Both problems can be uncomfortable and embarrassing. Although chemical-laden products such as cortisone may temporarily reduce the symptoms of the inflammation, they can further irritate the skin and possibly extend the duration of the condition because they don't treat the underlying source of the problem.

Internally and externally, coconut oil can be used as an all-natural, safe, and effective aid to psoriasis and eczema. Coconut oil's lauric acid contains anti-inflammatory properties that help to relieve the redness and itchiness of these conditions. In addition, lauric acid's antibacterial, antifungal, antiviral, and antimicrobial agents help improve your skin's health and appearance.

FOR INTERNAL AID, USE:

1 to 3 tablespoons of coconut oil

Ingest daily alone or in food to safeguard your skin from further irritation.

FOR TOPICAL RELIEF, USE:

As much coconut oil as needed

Apply to irritated areas of skin to soften scaly patches.

You'll see improvement in a matter of days—perhaps even hours. Not only does coconut oil provide quick relief, it can help to prevent eczema and psoriasis and their unpleasant symptoms forever!

Making these lifestyle changes may also improve your psoriasis or eczema:

■ Limit alcohol consumption.
■ Cut down on sugar in your diet.
■ Reduce exposure to sunlight and conditions that dry out the skin.

You may also want to add apple cider vinegar to your regime. Pour ½ cup of apple cider vinegar and ½ cup of water into a bowl and mix. Soak a clean towel in the solution and apply the wet towel directly to the affected area of skin for 30 minutes.

67. APPLY THE PERFECT P.M. MOISTURIZER

At night, your skin gets a chance to re-generate and refresh. While you sleep, your sensitive skin isn't exposed to the elements or to dirt and grime that might clog your pores. Take advantage of the hours you spend sleeping to moisturize your face with coconut oil—it can help improve the texture, evenness of tone, pore size, and luminosity of your skin in just a matter of days.

With thousands of moisturizing creams and lotions available, it can be difficult to determine which one is right for you. What if you knew that you could have a wrinkle reducer, an intensive acne combatant, a skin-tone corrector, and deep moisturizing treatment all in one? You can with coconut oil! Coconut oil provides a number of skin benefits that not only help improve your skin's quality with moisturizers, but also its appearance with wrinkle-fighting, anti-aging protection from the collagen-restoring capric acid.

Apply coconut oil to your skin before you sleep by soaking a cotton ball in the liquefied oil and applying it evenly to your entire face. Allow the oil to absorb for at least 5 minutes before you go to bed to ensure the coconut oil won't rub off on pillows or sheets, and then drift into slumber knowing your face is being treated with the oil's beneficial, naturally occurring phytochemicals and unique properties of lauric and capric acids that will help you keep your youthful glow as you age beautifully.

PORE-CLOGGING POTIONS

Before you coat your face with the latest skin cream designed to help the health and appearance of the skin on your face, you should be aware that many of these creams contain elements that can block pores and lead to blemishes. Coconut oil's lauric and capric acids help remove the environmental toxins that settle in the pores of your face throughout the day, and also open your pores, allowing them to "breathe" once the oil has dried. By opting for all-natural coconut oil as your go-to nighttime treatment, you can rest easy and live blemish free.

68. MAKE A FABULOUS FACE MASK

If you find yourself troubled by oily skin, dry skin, acne breakouts, skin discoloration, or even fine lines and wrinkles, you can benefit greatly from using a simple facial mask once per week. Although commercially available masks claim to cleanse, restore moisture, or provide age-defying results, most use synthetic additives to achieve those results. Coconut oil, when used as the base of your face mask, offers cleansing, moisturizing, and anti-aging benefits due to its lauric acid. Combine it with natural ingredients you have in your pantry and refrigerator, and you can quickly, easily, and inexpensively create your unique facial mask right in your own home.

> **YOU CAN TAILOR THIS MASK RECIPE BY ADDING INGREDIENTS FROM THE FOLLOWING LIST TO SUIT YOUR SKIN'S NEEDS:**

Start with 2 tablespoons of coconut oil as your base, then combine:

- **Oily skin:** 2 teaspoons apple cider vinegar—it dries up excess oil without drying out skin
- **Dry skin:** 2 teaspoons honey and 1 teaspoon almond milk—they help restore moisture and improve the skin's ability to retain moisture
- **Puffy skin:** 2 tablespoons espresso and 2 tablespoons natural cocoa, plus 1 tablespoon honey (dry skin) or lemon juice (oily skin)— espresso and cocoa's naturally occurring phytochemicals help to relieve inflammation
- **Discoloration:** ½ cup fresh pumpkin pulp—the antioxidants contained in pumpkin pulp help to restore proper pigmentation levels of the skin, and help reduce blotchiness and discoloration

After you combine the ingredients, apply the mask to your face and allow the mask to set for 10 to 15 minutes before washing and moisturizing as usual. You can repeat the mask treatments as often as daily, and as sparingly as weekly.

> **THE RIGHT TYPE OF APPLE CIDER VINEGAR FOR MAXIMUM BENEFITS**

Select apple cider vinegar that is unfiltered, unpasteurized, organic, and non-GMO. This enzyme-rich variety of vinegar will provide you with a number of amazing benefits to help prevent illness and improve health.

69. EXFOLIATE YOUR FACE GENTLY

Exfoliating your face removes dead skin cells that can make your complexion look less than luminous. Without this layer of dead cells forming a barrier on your skin, your moisturizer can work better, too. Instead of using products that contain chemicals and harsh abrasives, opt for natural solutions that safeguard your skin and improve its appearance at the same time. Combine coconut oil with all-natural ingredients that maximize your skin's health and improve its tone, elasticity, and clarity to create a gentle facial exfoliant right in your own home—for a fraction of the price of commercial products.

COMBINE THE FOLLOWING INGREDIENTS TO CREATE A GENTLE SCRUB THAT YOU CAN USE IN YOUR DAILY SKIN-CARE REGIMEN:

½ cup coconut oil
2 tablespoons brown sugar
⅛ cup pumpkin pulp
5 drops rosehip oil

Rinse your face thoroughly and apply a generous amount of the mixture to your face. Gently massage your skin. Be sure to not scrape your face with the brown sugar granules, as sugar can be abrasive when combined with rough movements or excessive pressure. Don't use white sugar; it's too abrasive. If you find the brown sugar to be too abrasive, allow the sugar to dissolve somewhat in the coconut oil before combining with the additional ingredients and applying to your face. Rinse with warm water. Store any remaining mixture in an airtight container in a place that isn't exposed to sunlight.

Following the exfoliation, be sure to moisturize your skin with a teaspoon of coconut oil to smooth your skin and improve collagen production. Coconut oil's vitamins, minerals, phytochemicals, and lauric and capric acids promote health and fight off immunity-attacking bacteria, viruses, and illnesses that can damage your skin. Thus, coconut oil is the perfect base for gentle exfoliating scrubs. Plus you can be sure that you're not only improving the quality of your skin, but that your made-at-home product is safe enough to use as often as you please.

70. REPAIR "DISHPAN HANDS"

Cracked, dry skin is a common problem when you do work that requires your hands to get wet and then dried multiple times throughout the day. Steaming hot water, as is commonly used for washing dishes, exacerbates the problem (hence the name "dishpan hands"). Those dishes are not going to wash themselves, though. So, how can you safeguard your hands and still get the job done? Use coconut oil, of course, to keep your hands clean, free of dish grime, and moisturized.

TO PROTECT YOUR HANDS WITH COCONUT OIL, USE:

2 teaspoons of coconut oil, separated

Rub 1 teaspoon of the oil on your hands before washing dishes and another teaspoon after you've finished, to keep skin moisturized and healthy.

Excessive heat or cold, both in the water that you're using for cleaning and in the environment around you, plus harsh cleansers and repeated scrubbing can cause dishpan hands to quickly develop into sensitive, red, or even blistery hands that are not only uncomfortable but also unsightly. Coconut oil, with lauric acid and capric acid that act as cleaning agents and moisturizers, can save wear and tear on your hands. As a precautionary measure, rub coconut oil on your hands (front and back) prior to washing dishes. Apply oil to your hands again after you've finished to prevent dishpan hands from developing and keep your skin smooth and supple long after those dishes are done!

71. CARE FOR YOUR SKIN WITH COCONUT OIL BODY BALM

Harsh weather, sun exposure, illness, stress, poor diet, allergies, and aging all take a toll on your body—and your skin is often the first place to show signs of distress. Because your skin is your body's largest organ and your first line of defense against environmental elements, it's important to give it the best possible care. Coconut oil's medium-chain fatty acids lock in moisture and keep your skin free of inflammation, irritation, and dryness. The oil can also help to combat damage and speed your body's regenerative processes.

COMBINE THESE THERAPEUTIC OILS TO CREATE THIS LUXURIOUS COCONUT OIL BODY BALM:

1 cup coconut oil

2 teaspoons almond oil

2 drops lavender, clary sage, myrrh, calendula, balsam, or fennel essential oil

Apply this safe, homemade coconut oil body balm to your skin at least once per day. For optimal results, you can rub on the body balm in the morning following your shower, one time during the day to remoisturize your skin, and one final time before going to bed. This special blend of healing oils helps to keep your skin soft and youthful so that every square inch of your body is as healthy and beautiful as you've always dreamed it could be.

72. MAKE A SUGARY BODY SCRUB

Just as removing the dead skin cells on your face via exfoliation can enhance your youthful glow, exfoliating the rest of your body on a regular basis keeps your skin from looking drab or unhealthy. Dryness and dullness can result from the buildup of these dead skin cells. Fret not—these conditions can quickly be remedied with body scrubs that exfoliate dead skin cells, moisturize rough patches of skin, and improve your skin's radiance. Opt for a natural method that can live up to the expensive commercial scrubs, instead of using a product that may contain chemicals or harsh ingredients that irritate your skin rather than enlivening it.

You can utilize your trusty coconut oil as a base for a sugary body scrub that's effective, inexpensive, safe, and natural, using ingredients you may already have in your home. Coconut oil provides the moisture-rich base, brown sugar crystals scrub away dead skin cells, and essential oils enhance the radiance of your skin. In addition, this sweet scrub helps to heal abrasions and discolorations on your skin's surface, and locks in moisture for hours.

TO MAKE THIS FRAGRANT SUGARY BODY SCRUB, BLEND:

1 cup coconut oil

½ cup brown sugar

2 teaspoons honey

2 to 5 drops lavender, clary sage, myrrh, calendula, balsam, or fennel essential oil, or a blend of two or more oils

Use this body scrub in your shower, massaging your skin in circular motions and rinsing with warm water. After toweling off, the most beneficial moisturizing treatment you can use to retain your skin's health and glow is a simple slather of coconut oil.

Allow the coconut oil to absorb into your skin—it will keep your skin moisturized and free of redness, itchiness, or irritation. You'll smell nice, too.

73. HEAL CUTS FASTER

A laceration on your skin opens an accessible route to your underlying skin tissues and blood vessels that germs can quickly infiltrate. Your body works diligently at the site of the cut, trying to repair the wound and regenerate the skin cells necessary to close the cut. Coconut oil can help you minimize your body's workload and safeguard your skin from infection.

TO BOLSTER YOUR IMMUNE SYSTEM AND HELP IT FIGHT INFECTIONS, USE:

1 to 3 tablespoons of coconut oil

Consume daily, neat or in your food.

AS A TOPICAL AID, USE:

A small amount of coconut oil

Apply directly to the cut itself as well as the surrounding area.

The oil provides the affected area with protective antibodies and powerful restorative elements that result from its lauric acid, capric acid, vitamins, and minerals to aid in the skin's recovery. Although you can find a number of antibiotic, over-the-counter creams and ointments that claim to heal minor wounds, they are often loaded with chemicals that may cause unwanted reactions. The lactic acid in coconut oil contains antibacterial qualities that fight infection that can accompany skin lacerations. These naturally occurring properties protect skin and promote healing safely, with no unwanted side effects. Included in your daily regimen, coconut oil can be a powerful immunity-boosting addition to your lifestyle, limiting the possibilities of infection once you suffer a cut. Coconut oil also speeds healing time by promoting your body's existing healing capabilities.

FIRST AID FOR CHILDREN

Scrapes, cuts, and other "boo-boos" are common in children from the time they begin toddling. Instead of coating the wound with antibiotic ointment or alcohol, apply coconut oil—the natural, antibiotic, anti-inflammatory properties in its lauric acid help prevent infection and promote healing. Cover the wound at night for added protection.

74. PREVENT SKIN INFECTIONS

When you have a cut, a burn, or other skin injury, your system is forced to work overtime in order to heal the condition and restore the body to normal. If infection invades your body via an opening in the skin, a weakened immune system results. If your immune system is already impaired, you're more susceptible to bacterial or viral infections. Coconut oil's antibacterial and antifungal properties from lauric acid and capric acid help prevent infection when you apply the oil topically to the site of a wound or lesion. When ingested in a daily dose of 1 to 3 tablespoons, coconut oil's lauric acid strengthens your immune system, enabling your body to ward off infections. Here's a great way to protect against infection by combining coconut oil's immunity-boosting properties with the vitamins and minerals in healthy green veggies.

THIS RECIPE FOR A GREENS GALORE SMOOTHIE MAKES 3 CUPS.

1 tablespoon coconut oil
1 cup coconut milk, separated
½ cup frozen mangoes
1 cup spinach
1 cup kale

Place coconut oil into a high-speed blender.

Add ½ cup of coconut milk and frozen mangoes. Blend until emulsified.

Add spinach and kale to the blender, and blend on high while adding the remaining ½ cup of coconut milk until all ingredients are well blended.

75. FIGHT ATHLETE'S FOOT

Athlete's foot is an uncomfortable condition that results from a fungus forming on the foot and between the toes. When your feet are subjected to wet, warm conditions—as happens when moisture and sweat collect in your shoes and remain on your feet for extended periods of time—fungus can thrive. Coconut oil provides a safe, natural, and effective way to help keep your feet free of fungus and to reduce the discomfort of athlete's foot once it develops.

The antifungal property in coconut oil's lauric acid helps to ensure that your feet will remain fungus-free.

The lauric acid in coconut oil boosts your immune system to help safeguard your body from illnesses and conditions such as athlete's foot.

You can take preventative measures to ensure that the fungus doesn't get a foothold, including:

- Keeping your feet dry (as much as possible)
- Airing out your shoes after you remove them
- Using powder on your feet when they'll be exposed to moist, enclosed conditions such as wet shoes
- Keeping your feet thoroughly clean

76. SOOTHE AND MOISTURIZE DRY FEET

Your feet take a beating every day, supporting your entire weight on a small surface area. Your ankles and heels are especially susceptible to dry skin and irritation from your shoes. If you go barefoot or wear minimally protective shoes such as flip-flops, you expose your feet to a number of environmental conditions that can contribute to dryness, cracked skin, and irritation. Unsightly and uncomfortable, dry skin on your feet can become an embarrassing condition.

In order to prevent dry skin on your feet and the painful symptoms that can result, you should:

■ Regularly remove the dry skin on your feet—especially your heels—using a pumice stone and the "Sugary Body Scrub" described earlier in this chapter.
■ Moisturize your feet daily.
■ Minimize the exposure to harmful elements and harsh conditions in the environment that can contribute to dry skin.

Coconut oil's quality moisturizing properties can improve the quality of the skin on your feet. Apply the oil topically to help repair cracked skin and speed the healing time of wounds. With its medium-chain fatty acids producing the powerful lauric acid's antibacterial, antiviral, antifungal, and antimicrobial benefits, coconut oil can also promote foot health by defending against germs that can cause infection. Coconut oil's anti-inflammatory properties can also reduce swelling and stimulate blood circulation to the feet. In addition to using coconut oil topically to prevent dry skin, consume 1 to 3 tablespoons daily, by itself or in your food, to improve your overall well-being. You'll soon be able to wear shoes that show off your healthy feet without embarrassment.

Chapter 4
HAIR AND BODY CARE

Peruse a popular women's magazine. Wander down the aisles of your local drugstore. You may feel overwhelmed by the incredible number of personal care products that promise a quick fix for everything from wrinkles to frizzy hair to discolored teeth. The beauty and personal care industry rakes in more than $250 billion globally each year. If you're like most people, you've probably fed the industry by purchasing hordes of jars, tubes, and bottles of stuff that promised to make you look better—many of which just clutter up your bathroom drawers or dresser top.

What would you say if I told you that you need only one product—that's right, just one—to handle everything? It might sound simplistic or even ridiculous that a single product—and an all-natural, inexpensive one at that—can address your many needs, but it's true. That miracle product is coconut oil. In this chapter, you'll discover twenty-four ways that coconut oil can stimulate hair growth, moisturize dry skin, minimize spider veins and cellulite, brighten your smile, and lots more. And the benefits don't stop there.

When you include coconut oil in your daily beauty and body care regimen, you'll not only improve your appearance, you'll improve your health and vitality, too, naturally and safely. Rather than forking out money on questionable products that at best offer a cover-up or temporary improvement, opt for a jar of extra virgin, organic coconut oil. You'll soon look and feel your best, not only on the surface but deep within as well.

77. DEFRIZZ HAIR

Dealing with frizzy hair is an annoying part of almost every curly-haired girl's life. Whether you have naturally frizz-prone hair or have self-induced the problem with the excessive use of products and treatments, taming your wild tresses into sleek submission doesn't have to be difficult, nor does it require a daily battle. Commercial defrizzing products often fail to deliver the desired results. They may leave hair excessively oily or greasy, or even further damage hair with chemical frizz-fighting serums. Luckily, coconut oil offers an outstanding way to improve the quality of your hair and remedy the frizzies safely, effectively, and naturally.

Depending upon the length of your hair, its texture, and the severity of damage (if any), the frequency and duration of your coconut oil treatments will vary. After one application, however, you will be able to determine how often you should repeat the process.

1. Fill a spray bottle with ½ cup of liquid coconut oil.
2. Prepare your hair by rinsing it thoroughly with water and towel drying it lightly to remove any excess water.
3. While your hair is damp, spray the coconut oil onto your hair until well saturated but not dripping.
4. Cover your hair with a shower cap or plastic wrap, allowing your body heat to improve the absorption of the oil into the hair strands.
5. Leave the oil on your hair for 1 to 2 hours before shampooing, conditioning, and styling as usual.

Not only will coconut oil smooth the frizzies, it will add shine and improve your hair's overall health.

78. FIGHT FRIZZ ON THE GO

After prepping and primping for an important meeting or big date, your image can be completely derailed by frizzy, unmanageable locks that look nothing like you planned. Humidity, heat, wind, and rain can wreak havoc on your tresses and cause frizz for even the most manageable hair. You can't control the weather, so what to do when you're trying to look your best but need to be prepared for the worst?

IF YOU'RE AWARE OF HIGH HUMIDITY OR RAIN IN THE FORECAST, TURN TO COCONUT OIL FOR A QUICK, NATURAL SOLUTION.

½ teaspoon of coconut oil for short hair and up to 1 teaspoon for long, thick hair

Evenly distribute the oil on the ends and throughout your hair prior to heat treating and styling, to prevent frizz before it starts.

Stash a mini-bottle of coconut oil in your purse, your car, or your desk drawer to treat those pesky flyaway strands and bouts of the frizzies any time they strike. Simply warm ¼ to ½ teaspoon of coconut oil in your hands and lightly apply it to your trouble areas. This effective, on-the-go frizz-fighter is natural and free of damaging chemicals, and leaves your hair smooth, shiny, and luxurious.

ADD ESSENTIAL OILS TO BOOST BENEFITS

To boost coconut oil's benefits and customize your hair treatment, try blending in a few drops of essential oil. Chamomile oil is good for dry, brittle hair, and an after-shampoo rinse of chamomile tea brings out highlights in blond hair. Lavender oil stimulates hair growth and helps ease the itching associated with dandruff. If your hair is oily, combine lemon oil with coconut oil or add lemon oil to your favorite shampoo.

79. STRENGTHEN HAIR

Long, lustrous locks are your crowning glory, but there is no magical pill, potion, or cream that delivers fast results to lengthen and strengthen your hair. A number of lifestyle habits can enhance or degrade the quality of your hair, so if your goal is to have long, healthy, beautiful tresses you should eat plenty of whole foods and healthy fats, while minimizing foods that are heavily processed or contain lots of preservatives. Because hair is made mostly of protein, it requires protein to grow strong; therefore, eating a diet that's rich in high-quality protein is essential.

In addition, a combination of apple cider vinegar and coconut oil can improve the texture, shine, and overall health of your hair. If you color your hair, heat-style it, perm it, or expose it to damaging chemicals such as chlorine or water-softening agents, you may need some extra TLC to keep your hair looking great. Even natural, untreated hair is exposed to dirt, pollution, and environmental toxins every day that can damage its health and deteriorate its strength. Try this "secret weapon":

1. Rinse your hair with apple cider vinegar to cleanse your hair of impurities.
2. Follow with a deep-conditioning application of coconut oil to restore and balance the natural, healthy oils in your hair and on your scalp. You can allow the coconut oil to set on your strands for one hour or up to two days, depending upon how dry your hair is.
3. Shampoo and condition as usual.

By performing this regimen at least once per week, you can boost your hair's health, strength, and appearance.

80. STIMULATE HAIR GROWTH

Whether you're trying to grow your hair longer or stimulate growth in areas of thinning hair, commercial products often fail to deliver the promised results. Additionally, these potions and lotions may be packed with harsh chemicals that can damage your hair or seep through your scalp and infiltrate your blood stream through the numerous veins that lie just below the skin of your scalp.

If you're seeking a safe, natural way to stimulate hair growth, look no further than coconut oil. Its moisturizing properties help to maximum moisture retention at the base of the hair shaft. Coconut oil also stimulates collagen production, due to its lauric acid and capric acid that combine to promote the regeneration of skin cells and hair follicle production, which can help improve hair quality and encourage new hair growth.

USE THIS SIMPLE PROCEDURE TO OPTIMIZE HAIR GROWTH BY PROTECTING THE NEW HAIR'S STRUCTURE AND DELIVERING POWERFUL PHYTOCHEMICALS AND VITAMIN E TO THE SCALP:

½ cup of coconut oil

Massage oil into your scalp and hair. Allow the oil to be absorbed for 1 to 3 hours, or up to a day if you have the time. Rinse, then shampoo and condition as usual. Repeat the process every 1 to 3 days to maximize results.

To support this topical application, consume 1 to 3 tablespoons of coconut oil per day. This enhances hair growth by enabling your body to better absorb the vitamins and minerals needed to maintain hair health.

CAN YOUR PONYTAIL DAMAGE YOUR HAIR?

Yes! Surprisingly enough, studies have shown that when the hair is repeatedly pulled into a ponytail, the strands of the hair are exposed to more stretching and breaking. Wet hair, which is weaker than dry, is more prone to damage.

81. DEFY DANDRUFF

To relieve dandruff, you have to attack the problem at its source: a dry scalp. Medicated shampoos available through prescription or over the counter can be packed with harsh chemicals and oily lotions that either exacerbate a dry scalp or leave your hair feeling greasy. By combining natural coconut oil with a relaxing massage technique, you can relieve yourself of dandruff while simultaneously treating your scalp to a number of other benefits that we've already discussed.

TO GAIN THESE BENEFITS WITH EASY APPLICATIONS THAT TAKE ONLY MINUTES, USE:

½ cup of coconut oil

Wet your hair and separate it into sections, making the scalp easily accessible. Apply oil at the base of the hair directly on the scalp, progressing through sections until the entire scalp is evenly saturated. Massage the oil into the scalp gently, using circular motions. Allow the oil to absorb into the scalp for up to 5 minutes before rinsing and shampooing as usual.

You can repeat the process as often as needed, but for optimal results, use this method daily until dandruff subsides. Repeat at least 2 to 3 times weekly for maintenance.

GET EXTRA BENEFITS FROM ESSENTIAL OILS

A number of essential oils can complement coconut oil in the fight against dandruff. Tea tree oil's antiseptic properties can help destroy bacteria on your scalp. Lavender, juniper, rosemary, ylang-ylang, and peppermint provide cleansing, purifying, and calming benefits. Blend about 5 to 10 drops of one of these oils—or a combination—into coconut oil and rub the mixture on your scalp. Leave it for about 5 minutes before rinsing and shampooing.

82. ADD SHINE TO HAIR

Most commercial products intended to add shine to your hair contain chemicals that develop a reflective film on the hair shaft. This appears to add shine, but the effect rinses away with just one, or maybe a few, washes—and those chemicals can leave your hair feeling dried out or damaged. If you're trying to restore a lustrous glow to your locks, you can enhance your hair's health with coconut oil to bring out natural shine and highlights without chemicals and additives.

Coconut oil's naturally occurring, deep-moisturizing properties due to high concentrations of lauric and capric acids not only treat hair with the nutrients necessary to achieve a healthy glow, but also help your scalp develop collagen to strengthen hair from root to tip. In this case, the most effective treatment you can find is also the safest.

1. In the shower, apply coconut oil to your wet hair.
2. Allow the oil to set for 3 to 5 minutes.
3. Rinse and shampoo as usual.

4. Follow with your regular styling method.

To improve the quality of your hair's health and safeguard it from the elements it is exposed to every day, use this application 1 to 2 times per week. You hair will shine from within, not merely with a synthetic film.

PROTEIN PROTECTION FOR YOUR HAIR

A study published in the March–April 2003 issue of *Journal of Cosmetic Science* tested coconut oil, mineral oil, and safflower oil to see which offered the best benefits to hair. Researchers found that only coconut oil reduced protein loss in hair, thereby improving the quality of damaged hair and preventing future damage. What's the secret? "Coconut oil, being a triglyceride of lauric acid (principal fatty acid), has a high affinity for hair proteins and . . . is able to penetrate inside the hair shaft."

83. PREVENT SPLIT ENDS

You'll notice the title of this section is "Prevent Split Ends," not "Repair Split Ends," because once a hair splits, it is absolutely impossible to reunite the hair strand. With the right techniques, however, you can prevent split ends before they start, allowing your hair to grow longer, faster, and without frizz. The bad news is that split strands will continue to split up the hair shaft until you cut your hair above the portion where the splitting occurred. On a lighter note, ridding your hair of the dry, discolored, and unmanageable ends can revive the health of your hair quickly and give it a better appearance.

To prevent split ends in the future, begin by improving your hair-care regimen and maintaining a healthy lifestyle. Your diet, too, contributes tremendously to the quality of your hair. Try these things to promote healthy hair free of split ends:

- Apply ½ teaspoon of coconut oil to the ends of your hair after a shower to nourish and moisturize the tips. The phytochemicals in coconut oil that provide a unique and sensual texture are the same properties responsible for moisturizing strands.

- Avoiding brushing your hair when wet—it's most fragile at this stage.

- Minimize chemical treatments, such as coloring and perming, that can damage the hair shaft or root.

- Allow your hair to dry somewhat before applying heat during the styling process.

- Eat a diet rich in whole foods and avoid processed foods that are high in sugar and unhealthy fat. Because hair is made up mostly of protein, be sure to get plenty of high-quality protein in your diet.

- Once or twice weekly, use the regimen described in the earlier entry "Strengthen Hair" to ensure that your hair receives adequate moisture.

84. EAT COCONUT ITALIAN KABOBS TO NOURISH YOUR HAIR

Because your diet is the most important factor in your hair's health, you'll want to pay special attention to the foods you eat in order to improve the strength, shine, and overall quality of your tresses. The nutrients you get from a diet rich in whole foods and free of processed, sugary foods will quickly show benefits in your hair, skin, and the rest of your body. This beautifully colored dish combines foods from the Italian diet—tomatoes, olives, spinach, basil, and mozzarella—in a convenient kabob that your friends and family will love.

DRESS THESE COLORFUL ITALIAN KABOBS WITH COCONUT OIL HERB DRESSING AND SERVE 8 WITH THIS EASY, HEALTHY RECIPE.

1 cup spinach leaves (48 leaves)
16 black olives
1 cup basil leaves (48 leaves)
16 cherry tomatoes
16 mini mozzarella balls
½ cup coconut oil, melted
2 tablespoons *herbes de Provence*
8 kabob sticks

On each kabob stick, spear 3 spinach leaves, 1 olive, 3 basil leaves, 1 cherry tomato, and 1 mozzarella ball; repeat to make two sequences on each kabob.

In a small measuring cup, combine coconut oil and *herbes de Provence* and mix well.

Drizzle kabobs with oil and herb dressing, turning periodically to ensure equal coating throughout.

Because your hair is made mainly of protein, you may want to increase the amount of protein in this recipe by adding chicken, shrimp, or beef to the basic recipe. Cube and cook the meat prior to skewering it.

85. WHITEN TEETH

Did you know that most of the stains and discoloration that occur on teeth can be easily removed and prevented with simple, inexpensive at-home treatments? You can enjoy coffee, tea, and red wine without developing the yellowish or grayish discoloration that often results—and without the chemicals contained in popular, commercial teeth-whitening products.

COMBINE THREE SIMPLE INGREDIENTS TO BRUSH AWAY STAINS, WHITEN TEETH, AND PREVENT FUTURE STAINS. IT WORKS QUICKLY—AND YOU DON'T HAVE TO REFRAIN FROM EATING AND DRINKING FOR HOURS BEFORE AND AFTER THE PROCEDURE.

1 teaspoon coconut oil

1 teaspoon apple cider vinegar (the unfiltered, unpasteurized, organic version)

1 teaspoon hydrogen peroxide

1 tablespoon water

Combine all the ingredients. Sip the concoction; swish throughout your mouth and over your teeth for a minimum of 1 minute and up to 5 minutes. Spit out the mixture and brush teeth as usual. You can repeat the process as often as necessary throughout the day to brighten your teeth and safeguard your pearly whites.

Other products improve your teeth's appearance by using leaching methods to enhance color. However, the three ingredients recommended here combine to remove stains by restoring their natural, healthy sheen while also illuminating their color and preventing future stains. You'll see results after only a few simple, inexpensive treatments.

WHITEN TEETH WITH APPLE CIDER VINEGAR

The enzymes (referred to as "the mother") in apple cider vinegar help to remove stains caused by bacteria, safeguarding your teeth from deposits that cause unsightly discoloration. By daily swishing this bacteria-fighting product in your mouth, you can be sure you're reaping optimum benefits . . . naturally.

86. "PULL" BACTERIA FROM YOUR MOUTH

Even though "pulling" is growing in popularity, most people are still unaware of the method or why people do it. Pulling is an ancient Indian therapy that involves swishing oils in the mouth for a brief time, allowing the oil to pull bacteria and germs from the gums, tongue, and teeth. You literally spit the harmful elements out of your mouth, thereby ridding your body of germs and impurities that could cause infections. In past centuries, a variety of oils were used for the pulling method, but recently coconut oil has become one of the most popular due to lauric acid's potent germ-killing property.

TO PERFORM PULLING, USE:

1 tablespoon of coconut oil

Swish the coconut oil all around your mouth—teeth and gums, under the tongue—for 15 to 20 minutes. Spit the oil from your mouth into a sink and rinse the sink thoroughly. Immediately after spitting out the coconut oil, brush your teeth thoroughly. Repeat the process daily.

The mouth contains both good and bad bacteria. Coconut oil is one of the only oils that attacks the bad while promoting the growth of the good. Pulling with coconut oil helps to preserve the health of your mouth and safeguard teeth, gums, and tongue from infections that can result from plaque buildup and bad bacteria. Pulling with coconut oil can also improve the appearance of your teeth and gums by removing stains and preventing redness and irritation around the gums. (See the entry "Whiten Teeth" in this chapter for more information.)

87. SWITCH TO A NATURAL DEODORANT

Concerns about a possible link between the chemicals in deodorants/antiperspirants and breast cancer could be enough to make you switch to a natural product. Perhaps synthetic fragrances and other additives irritate your skin. Did you know that you can use coconut oil as a deodorant? Not only can the oil keep your armpits odor-free, it moisturizes your skin to help keep your armpits free of flakes, chafing, itching, and unsightly bumps.

Although many people neglect moisturizing their underarms, it is important to keep this sensitive skin moisturized just as you do the other parts of your body. Coconut oil not only softens your skin, its antibacterial, antifungal properties—inherent in lauric acid—kill bacteria and germs that can thrive in the armpits and cause body odor. The oil can also help heal small nicks that result from shaving.

Scoop up a teaspoon of solidified coconut oil and apply it to your underarm areas evenly. Your body's natural heat will cause the oil to melt and supply your underarms with a healthy dose of moisturizing-packed, bacteria-fighting agents that will keep you smelling fresh all day and night. Be sure to allow the coconut oil to fully dry before dressing, as excess oil may cause slight discoloration or oil stains on your clothing.

SYNTHETIC FABRICS INCREASE ODOR

Clothing made of synthetic materials can increase body odor by preventing air from reaching your armpits and trapping bacteria. This is especially true of fabrics used in athletic clothing, which are designed with tiny holes to wick away sweat. Those micro-holes are the perfect breeding ground for bacteria that can make you and your clothing stink. Instead of manmade fibers, wear cotton and other natural materials—you'll feel more comfortable, too.

88. ENHANCE EYELASHES

Your eyelashes have a very important role to play. They protect your eyes from dirt and other particulate matter in the environment that could cause irritation or damage. Of course, they also highlight the beauty of your eyes, just as a decorative frame enhances a painting. Because your eyes are so incredibly important, you don't want to subject them to just any old product—especially one full of chemicals that might harm your eyes. Err on the side of safety with this all-natural recipe that encourages lash growth.

USE THIS AROMATIC CLEANSING CONCOC-
TION TO REMOVE GRIME AND BUILDUP
FROM YOUR LASHES WHILE NOURISHING
AND CONDITIONING THEM WITH HEALTH-
PROMOTING PROPERTIES:

1 tablespoon coconut oil
1 teaspoon lemon juice

1 drop lavender oil

Thoroughly clean out a mascara tube and the brush. Combine all the ingredients in the clean tube. Dip the clean mascara brush into the mixture and apply to the lashes evenly. Apply 1 to 3 times daily, especially at night before bed.

Coconut oil combats microbes and stimulates growth. Astringent lemon juice provides cleansing properties. Lavender oil contains phytochemicals that can improve the growth of your lashes—and it smells nice, too. The unique blend doesn't just enhance your eyes' appearance temporarily, it can help make your eyelashes thicker, longer, and lovelier than ever. Be careful to avoid getting the concoction *in* your eyes, as the lemon juice can burn.

89. REMOVE MAKEUP NATURALLY

The most effective tool for taking off oil-based makeup is an oil-based remover. Some makeup removers contain chemicals that can actually damage your eyes, clog your pores, or irritate the skin of your face; therefore, they are not the best option for taking off your makeup at the end of the day. What you want instead is a makeup remover that not only cleans your face, but also contributes to the health and vitality of your skin. Coconut oil gently cleanses your skin and eyelashes, while also moisturizing your skin, safely and naturally.

THIS NATURAL CLEANSER, WITH THE ANTI-BACTERIAL PROPERTIES OF LAURIC ACID, CLEARS YOUR FACE OF POSSIBLE BACTERIA, DIRT, AND GRIME.

Coconut oil as needed

Soak a cotton ball in liquefied oil. Apply a thin coating of the oil to your face, eyelids, and lashes. Rinse with warm water to remove makeup and any dirt or bacteria that has deposited on your face throughout the day.

Additionally, coconut oil restores a healthy glow to your skin with circulation-improving properties from its lauric acid and collagen-promoting capric acid. Use the following method to remove your makeup safely and to improve your skin's health and appearance in the process. You can safely use coconut oil as often as needed to remove makeup and to brighten your complexion in the process.

After removing your makeup, you can opt to use the recipes in "Exfoliate Your Face Gently" and "Make a Fabulous Face Mask" in Chapter 3 to nourish your skin further. Apply a small amount of coconut oil to your face before you start your day and before you head to bed to improve the texture and overall health of your skin.

90. ENJOY A MOISTURIZING BATH

Almost 3,000 years ago, the Greek physician Hippocrates touted the healthful benefits of bathing. In *The Scent Trail*, Celia Lyttelton quotes him as recommending "the way to health is to have an aromatic bath and scented massage every day." Throughout history, people around the world have flocked to sites renowned for their healing waters. Even today, millions of people look forward to their stress-reducing, relaxing baths that allow them to soak away daily cares in warm, soothing waters. Although the simple act of taking a bath can be enough to keep your stress at bay—as Hippocrates proposed—you can add to the enjoyment of your bath time by adding a healthy, moisturizing dose of coconut oil to your bathwater.

PUT IN SOME FRAGRANT ESSENTIAL OILS, SUCH AS LAVENDER, MYRRH, OR SANDALWOOD, TO REV UP THE RELAXING BENEFITS AND MAKE YOUR BATH EVEN BETTER.

½ to 1 cup coconut oil
Several drops of your favorite essential oil

Add oils to warm water in your bathtub. Sit and relax in the tub for 15 to 30 minutes, reaping maximum benefits from the intense moisturizing capabilities from the naturally occurring vitamin E and phytochemicals of the coconut oil.

Coconut oil's medium-chain fatty acids help to stimulate blood circulation and minimize the appearance of cellulite. The quickly absorbed, moisture-rich oil helps to eliminate dry patches of skin—and the oil's tropical aroma provides comfort and relaxation when added to bathwater.

91. LOVE YOUR LIP BALM

Cold weather, too much sun, and dry conditions can cause your lips to chap, crack, bleed, or become infected. Any products you apply to your lips to soothe them can easily be ingested, so when safeguarding your lips' health, follow this simple rule: Don't put anything on your lips that you wouldn't eat. I don't know about you, but I certainly wouldn't nosh on anything unless I knew how it was made and what it contained. Luckily, coconut oil does double duty as the best moisturizing, chap preventative available and as a natural aid for dry, cracked lips.

SIMPLY APPLY THE OIL IN ITS LIQUID OR SOLID STATE TO YOUR LIPS. OR, IF YOU PREFER, USE:

Coconut oil in its liquefied state, as needed
An empty tube of your old lip balm to hold the coconut oil

Rinse the tube thoroughly, pour in coconut oil, and refrigerate for at least an hour.

Now you have the perfect all-natural lip balm to help soothe chapping, prevent infection, and beautify your lips. Keeping the tube stored in a cool, dark place that is consistently 75°F or cooler will help maintain the coconut oil's solid state. Many varieties of commercial lip balm contain chemicals and synthetic fragrances or flavoring that can do more harm than good. Coconut oil, however, is packed with essential nutrients (including lauric and capric acids, and vitamin E) that protect your lips from environmental factors that can cause irritation, dryness, and blisters. Coconut oil is safe enough to consume on a regular basis. It also improves the health and appearance of your lips after just a few simple applications.

92. GET A SMOOTHER SHAVE WITH COCONUT CREAM

With moisturizing benefits galore, coconut oil is an ideal shaving cream, gentle and safe enough for your face, underarms, legs, even your bikini area. Not only does its lauric acid moisturize your skin and safeguard it from nicks and cuts that often occur while shaving, coconut oil also boosts your skin's health long after you've finished shaving. Whether you're tackling the thickest of men's beards or the most sensitive, feminine places that see no sunshine, coconut oil can help you achieve the perfect shave without redness, inflammation, or ingrown hairs. The lauric acid provided by coconut oil reduces inflammation of the skin while helping to fend off infections with its antibacterial, antiviral, and antimicrobial properties. The oil's capric acid components contain collagen-building and cell-regenerating properties that can improve the skin's overall appearance.

WHIPPING UP A QUICK BATCH OF COCONUT OIL SHAVING CREAM IS EASY. THE SLICK OIL LETS YOUR RAZOR GLIDE ALONG A SMOOTH SURFACE, PREVENTING ABRASION, AND DELIVERS MUCH-NEEDED MOISTURE TO HELP KEEP YOUR SKIN FREE OF DRY PATCHES.

Coconut oil as needed
Immersion blender

Insert the immersion blender into a container of coconut oil. Blend or whip at high speed for about a minute—the coconut oil forms a creamy version of itself that easily spreads on your skin for the perfect shave each and every time. Store the whipped oil in an airtight container in a cabinet or dark area that is 75°F or cooler for up to one week.

Unlike commercial shaving creams and gels, coconut oil's antibacterial and antimicrobial benefits also help to keep your skin safe from dirt and germs that settle on the skin's surface. Its collagen-building elements help to restore skin health and rejuvenate skin cells—just one more benefit that separates coconut oil from other products.

93. MINIMIZE SPIDER VEINS

Unsightly and sometimes uncomfortable, spider veins appear as purple, red, green, or deep blue lines that create a spider-web appearance just beneath the skin's surface. Although they pose no real health threat, they mar the appearance of the skin on your legs. The all-natural healing properties of coconut oil have given some women relief from spider veins. Try this simple two-step approach:

1. Warm coconut oil and apply it topically to the site of spider veins.
2. Consume 1 to 3 tablespoons of coconut oil per day.

The anti-inflammatory properties in coconut oil help to alleviate the inflammation that can occur beneath the skin as a result of restricted blood flow or excessive pressure and lead to spider veins. Applied topically to the skin, the oil soothes the inflamed areas to help return the veins to their original state. Coconut oil's lauric acid also improves blood flow, blood health, and circulation; this helps to reduce the appearance of spider veins by infiltrating the areas and relieving the veins of possible blockages. Chemicals injected into the veins may reduce the appearance of spider veins, and topical creams and dyes can mask the issue, but they often include questionable ingredients or uncomfortable processes. With coconut oil, you'll soon gain relief from spider veins and help prevent them from occurring in the future—without the pain or side effects that can accompany commercial procedures and creams that promise to eliminate spider veins.

IMPROVE YOUR CIRCULATION

Spider veins are often a sign of poor circulation. By getting more exercise on a regular basis, you may be able to prevent or reduce the prevalence of spider veins. Low-impact activities such as walking, swimming, bicycling, and yoga are good ways to increase circulation without putting excess stress on your body. Also, elevating your feet for periods of time throughout the day and keeping your feet and legs warm can be beneficial. Taking regular hot baths can help, too.

94. REDUCE THE APPEARANCE OF CELLULITE

Few people have anything nice to say about cellulite. Referred to as "skin dimpling," "crater skin," and just plain "fat," cellulite seems to plague almost every segment of the population, even skinny folks. Indiscriminate in terms of gender, height, weight, or level of fitness, cellulite attacks the stomach, thighs, and arms of genetically predisposed people. Coconut oil's unique, medium-chain fatty acids can actually speed the body's fat-burning potential and reduce the appearance of cellulite. (See "Increase Fat Loss" in Chapter 1 for more information.)

TO PERFORM SKIN BRUSHING (ALSO KNOWN AS "DRY-BRUSHING"), USE:

Coconut oil as needed
A natural-hair brush (soft bristles)

Apply coconut oil to the skin, then brush skin with a soft-bristle, natural-hair brush, using an upward motion. Do this for 10 minutes, 1 to 3 times daily.

TO ENCOURAGE YOUR BODY'S FAT-BURNING CAPABILITIES, USE:

1 to 3 tablespoons of coconut oil

Ingest the oil daily, alone or in food. Because cellulite is directly associated with the enlargement or engorgement of fat cells beneath the skin, increasing your intake of healthy dietary fat (such as the unique medium-chain fatty acids provided by coconut oil) can actually speed the body's fat-burning potential and reduce your overall body-fat percentage, resulting in a lower incidence of cellulite.

Cellulite is believed to occur when fat cells in the form of a honeycomb striation get pushed to the surface of the skin by excess fat deposits beneath the skin's surface. A number of contributing factors can exacerbate the appearance of cellulite; although genetics play a major part, certain lifestyle issues can contribute to the problem:

- A poor diet heavy in processed foods
- Smoking
- Excessive alcohol consumption
- A sedentary lifestyle

In addition to including coconut oil in your daily regimen, making some lifestyle changes can help you see dramatic results in as little as thirty days.

95. RELIEVE COLD SORES

Cold sores that occur around and inside the mouth are the result of the herpes simplex 1 virus, which is thought to be present in more than two-thirds of the U.S. population. This virus has shown to respond well to oral medications prescribed by physicians, as well as creams and ointments that improve the condition of the cold sore—though powerful antiviral drugs and treatments can cause discomfort for some people. Coconut oil, however, with its powerful, naturally occurring antiviral properties inherent in lauric acid, can help to relieve the embarrassment and discomfort of cold sores naturally, without any chemicals or painful applications.

AS AN INTERNAL PREVENTATIVE AND AID, USE:

1 to 3 tablespoons of coconut oil

Consume daily. Increase the dose up to double that amount when cold sores appear.

By ingesting the coconut oil, you can provide your body with immunity-boosting antiviral agents that can help to fight the virus within the body and alleviate the symptoms that result externally.

AS A TOPICAL OINTMENT, USE:

Coconut oil as needed

Apply directly to the site of a cold sore with a cotton ball multiple times a day and before bed. Do not reintroduce the cotton ball to the coconut oil once it has been in contact with the cold sore, to avoid contaminating the oil.

Without side effects, medications, or chemicals, coconut oil has been receiving more attention every year as the perfect antiviral application for reducing the incidence of the herpes simplex 1 virus in adults and children as well.

COCONUT OIL AND HERPES

In a 2012 article for *Herpes Bulletin*, Miguel Gonzalez, MD, reported a study that tested coconut oil's effect on the herpes virus. The results? Coconut oil's lauric and capric acids "caused a 100,000 fold reduction in the virus." Dr. Gonzalez also pointed out in the article that two often-prescribed medications for herpes reduced symptoms, whereas "coconut oil [has] the ability to actually destroy the herpes virus, and also prevent secondary bacterial or fungal herpes infections."

96. STIMULATE NAIL GROWTH

In order to develop strong, healthy nails that are able to grow long without breaking, splitting, or peeling, you have to feed your body the nutrients it needs and pay attention to the environments to which you subject your nails. Exposing them to excessive water, harsh weather, and chemicals (as commonly occurs when washing dishes) can undermine the strength and growth of your nails. But protecting your nails alone may not be enough.

Stimulating nail growth requires internal as well as external methods. Coconut oil not only provides phytochemicals and vitamin E needed for proper body system functioning, but also aids in the absorption of these nutrients.

- A dose of 1 to 3 tablespoons of coconut oil consumed daily can help improve the quality and growth of your nails from the inside out.
- To strengthen your nails even more, soak them in coconut oil for 5 minutes before bed. Pat them dry, but don't wash off the oil. Instead, allow your nails and the surrounding skin to absorb the oil throughout the night.
- Massage your nails throughout the day with coconut oil to keep them free of dirt and to fight germs that can interfere with nail growth and health.

A diet comprised of whole foods that provide your body with calcium, magnesium, silica, and other essential nutrients can aid hair and nail growth, too. And because your nails are made up of protein, make sure to eat plenty of high-quality protein. Eliminate foods that are nutrient-void and provide little or no value, and that may actually inhibit the absorption and utilization of existing nutrients your body needs for proper nail growth.

97. DRESS UP YOUR SALAD WITH COCONUT OIL

As you've learned from reading this book, consuming coconut oil daily can bring health benefits in every area of your life. But just eating a couple spoonfuls of the oil every day can get boring—that's why I've also included a number of tantalizing recipes and easy ways to include coconut oil in your food. This Tropical Island Salad Dressing is loaded with nutrients and all the many benefits of coconut oil. Drizzle it over mixed greens for a salubrious, summertime treat—you may also want to add a sprinkling of bacon bits for extra protein. Combine it with rice and serve cold on a bed of spinach or arugula, or hot as a delightful side dish with fish or pork. Spoon over fish or shrimp to add a surprising burst of tropical flavor.

COCONUT OIL PROVIDES THE DELICIOUS BASE FOR THIS DRESSING, WHICH MAKES ABOUT 10 3-OUNCE SERVINGS.

¾ cup coconut oil

¼ cup pineapple juice

½ cup pineapple

½ cup macadamia nuts

Combine all ingredients in a high-speed blender. Blend until all ingredients are emulsified.

This sweet and nutty dressing is so versatile, you'll probably think of a dozen different ways to enjoy it. Try it over vanilla ice cream, or as a topping for white or yellow cake. Or, how about on pancakes instead of syrup?

98. BANISH BRUISES

Bruising appears when a trauma to the skin produces broken blood vessels that can appear as green, brown, purple, blue, or even black marks. Based on the intensity of the injury, the bruising that results can remain for days to weeks. You can improve the rate by which your body heals itself and minimize the appearance and duration of bruising with coconut oil. Not only can the anti-inflammatory properties found in the lauric acid produced by the oil's medium-chain fatty acids treat bruising after the fact, coconut oil can also prevent or reduce the severity of bruising prior to trauma.

Ingesting 1 to 3 tablespoons of coconut oil per day supports the body's blood flow and circulation, while providing anti-inflammatory properties that can reduce pain and swelling at the site. This also helps your body to quickly and efficiently repair areas of damage resulting from trauma, and to restore your skin's original appearance.

YOU CAN ALSO USE COCONUT OIL TOPICALLY TO SPEED THE REPAIR PROCESS FOLLOWING BRUISING AND SKIN DAMAGE:

1 teaspoon to 1 tablespoon of coconut oil

Apply directly to the skin and gently massage the area for 5 minutes multiple times per day.

This helps to redistribute the components of the broken blood vessels and make them more easily "carried away" in the blood stream for removal.

By consuming a diet rich in vitamins, minerals, and phytochemicals found in fruits and vegetables, you can improve your body's functioning and support the recovery process activated after a traumatic experience that causes bruising. Vitamins C and E, iron and magnesium, and a number of phytochemicals that act as potent antioxidants combine to speed recovery while also reducing the incidence and severity of bruising.

99. RELIEVE DIAPER RASH

The interior conditions of a baby's diaper are damp, airless, and (more often than not) soiled with urine and/or excrement. These conditions create the perfect environment for chafing and skin irritations, commonly known as diaper rash. Once a diaper rash develops, the enclosed wet and/or soiled conditions further exacerbate the issue and can lead to skin breaks or sores. The open skin resulting from these irritations can become a breeding ground for bacteria and germs.

Fortunately, the lauric acid produced by the medium-chain fatty acids found in coconut oil not only relieves the discomfort of diaper rash, it also moisturizes baby's sensitive skin with natural oils. Plus coconut oil's antibacterial, antifungal properties help to fight the growth of bacteria, microbes, fungi, and viruses that can irritate a baby's bottom.

If you see redness and irritation starting to develop in any part of the diaper area, bathe your baby in a mixture of warm water and coconut oil. Then coat the irritated area with coconut oil and allow your baby to enjoy an extended period of time without a diaper (at least one hour). As an ongoing preventative, apply a teaspoon of the oil (in its liquid or solid form) to your baby's bottom after bathing and between diaper changes to help keep her free of rashes, irritations, and infections. In addition, you'll want to check diapers regularly and remove waste and wetness as soon and as often as possible. Allowing fresh air to reach your baby's bottom regularly throughout the day can also help reduce the incidence of diaper rashes and minimize the chance of infection.

100. SOOTHE NURSING MOM'S NIPPLES

When you're nursing your baby, your body produces moisturizing oils from the ducts on your nipples. Although these natural moisturizers are intended to nourish the nipples and prevent dryness and cracking, some moms still suffer from discomfort. To help prevent uncomfortable conditions such as chafing and irritation that can arise from nursing, you can take some precautionary measures to protect your nipples.

Coconut oil can serve as the perfect, all-natural moisturizer—rub it on prior to and after nursing, as often as necessary, without fear of side effects for mother or baby. Here's an added bonus: Coconut oil's antibacterial, antiviral, and antimicrobial properties help safeguard mom and baby from possible infections. Additionally, coconut oil contains lauric acid, which is also present in breastmilk. Obviously, you'll want to avoid any type of lubricant that contains chemicals or fragrances that might harm baby's delicate system.

For even greater relief:

- At night, apply an ample amount of coconut oil to your nipples and the surrounding breast skin.
- Wear unrestrictive clothing around your chest to reduce discomfort.
- Allow your nipples to "breathe" after nursing by exposing them to air for at least 10 or 15 minutes.

THE BEST SOURCE OF NUTRITION FOR BABIES

Numerous studies, including two published in 2014 in the journal *Pediatrics*, show that children who have been breastfed are less likely to contract ear, throat, and sinus infections than children who were bottle fed. Furthermore, the studies found that six-year-olds who had been nursed as infants had fewer food allergies. The American Academy of Pediatrics advises mothers to nurse their babies for the first year of life.

INDEX

ABOUT THE AUTHOR

Britt Brandon is a Certified Personal Trainer and Certified Fitness Nutrition Specialist (certified by the International Sports Sciences Association, ISSA) who has enjoyed writing books focusing on clean eating and fitness for Adams Media for the past four years. In her time with Adams, she has published many books: *The Everything® Green Smoothies Book*, *The Everything® Eating Clean Cookbook*, *What Color Is Your Smoothie?*, *The Everything® Eating Clean Cookbook for Vegetarians*, *The Everything® Guide to Pregnancy Nutrition & Health*, *The Everything® Healthy Green Drinks Book*, and *Apple Cider Vinegar for Health*. As a competitive athlete, trainer, mom of three small children, and fitness and nutrition blogger on her own website (*www.ultimatefitmom.com*), Britt is well-versed in the holistic approaches to keeping one's self in top performing condition . . . and uses coconut oil daily, as an addition to drinks, smoothies, and food, as well as in many home remedies.